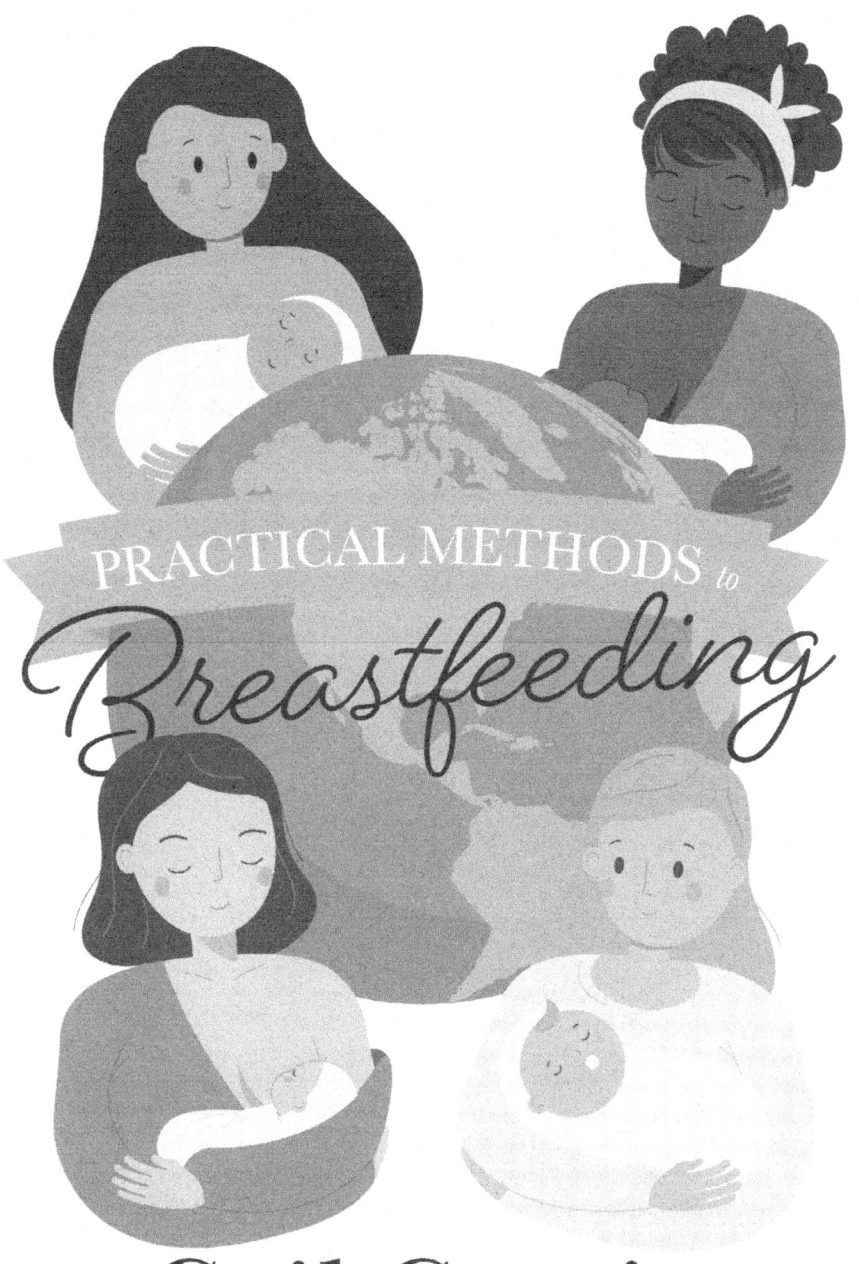

PRACTICAL METHODS *to*

Breastfeeding

Gail Curcio

Print ISBN: 978-1-09834-540-2

eBook ISBN: 978-1-09834-541-9

Table of Contents

Introduction... 1

Chapter 1: Mothers Deserve a Voice in the Feeding
Method for Their Babies 3

Chapter 2: Benefits of Breastfeeding and Reasons
Mothers Cannot Breastfeed 17

Chapter 3: Stimulation of the Breast Makes Milk.. 25

Chapter 4: Transition of Breast Milk from Birth to
Full Milk Production 30

Chapter 5: Breastfeeding Problems the First Two Weeks After Birth...... 36

Chapter 6: Comfort and Security Are Key to a Successful Latch-On..... 45

Chapter 7: Establishing a Schedule for Baby 59

Chapter 8: Possible Breastfeeding Problems and Treatments................... 63

Chapter 9: Returning to Work or School 87

Chapter 10: Diet and Medication in Breastfeeding...................................... 100

Chapter 11: Normal Physical Characteristics and
Care of the Newborn.. 104

Chapter 12: Weaning 115

References 119

Introduction

My name is Gail. I titled my book *Practical Methods to Breastfeeding because* I believe mothers need to be practical and realistic if they choose to breast-feed. When I assist mothers with breastfeeding, I ask them to revert to how our grandmothers fed their babies, watching for signs or cues their baby was hungry. All babies breastfed or bottle-fed will demonstrate feeding or hunger cues, such as fussiness, opening their eyes, hand-mouth activity, or playing with their tongue when they are hungry. Throughout my book, we will be discussing the use of your senses of seeing, hearing, and feeling to evaluate if your baby is hungry and ready to feed. My book is for you, the breastfeeding and bottle-feeding mother. I hope my ideas will help you to enjoy your feeding experience better. I think it is important to mention that I teach and write the way I learn through repetition. You will read the same information repeated multiple times for different situations. For example, I discuss various ways to stimulate your sleepy newborn to stay awake and breastfeed, which increases milk production. I will refer to babies in the male gender as he, him, or himself.

I cannot imagine how scared babies are at birth. We forget that they have been floating in warm amniotic fluid, hearing mothers' heartbeat, and feeling secure for 40 weeks. Your baby is born into bright lights, loud noises, a cold room, and placed on your chest skin-to-skin, which is encouraged to help him adjust to his new world or environment. Keeping your baby skin-to-skin will increase his comfort and security at the breast, which will increase breastfeeding success.

All of us have fears of the unknown, which is very scary. I believe breastfeeding is a fear of the unknown from negative perceptions mothers develop concerning breastfeeding, mainly because of the mother's information she hears from other mothers. With any fear of the unknown, increasing knowledge will decrease stress and anxiety. My goal is to lower your breastfeeding fears by providing you with step-by-step methods to increase your understanding of positioning and latching your baby onto the breast. I do not consider my book a textbook; it is a guide with explanations to help you breastfeed your baby. I compare my book to building a house, starting with the foundation. Each chapter of my book builds on the previous chapter, like building a home; you learn the steps of breastfeeding your baby. As you read and follow each chapter, you will be more prepared, less stressed, and more comfortable latching your baby onto your breast. Please remember you are not a super mom. Be patient and kind to yourself as you and your baby are learning to breastfeed.

Breastfeeding is a learned skill for both mom and baby. Mothers have to acquire breastfeeding information by taking classes; after the mother delivers her baby, she must trust that the hospital staff will continue to educate and assist her with breastfeeding. All mothers, breastfeeding or bottle-feeding, need support, guidance, education, assistance, and follow up. In my book, you will read about multiple reasons why you may need to supplement your baby. Supplementation means feeding your baby pumped milk or formula by way of a syringe or a bottle in the place of breastfeeding. In situations where supplementing your baby may be needed, keep an open mind. The health of your baby is the priority. The feeding method of breastfeeding, bottle-feeding, or a combination of both is the mother's decision.

Chapter 1:

Mothers Deserve a Voice in the Feeding Method for Their Babies

"Are you going to breastfeed?" Every mother is asked this question from conception, throughout her pregnancy, and after delivery. Mothers are pressured and almost forced to breastfeed, whether they want to or not. Mothers deserve a voice in their baby's feeding method, without criticism, degradation, or guilt.

Multiple mothers I have assisted with breastfeeding have made these and similar comments:

- "Giving my baby a pacifier will prevent my baby from breastfeeding."

- "I cannot bond with my baby if I don't breastfeed."

- "I am taking risks with my baby's health if I give my baby formula."

- "If I give my baby a bottle, he will never nurse."

"Do you need help latching your baby on the breast?" Mother's are not asked, "How do you want to feed your baby?" Mothers tell me they feel pushed to breastfeed. When mothers decide to bottle-feed and not to breastfeed, the nurses' and lactation consultants' responses in the hospital are negative. Some mothers have medical reasons they cannot breastfeed, or they do not want to breastfeed. Mothers who choose to bottle-feed their baby formula have asked me why their needs are not as important as those of a breastfeeding mother. Why do the needs of a breastfeeding mother appear more important than the needs of a bottle-feeding mother? Some hospitals are placing signs on breastfeeding mothers' cribs, stating, "My Mother Loves Me, She Is Breastfeeding. " This statement makes the bottle-feeding mothers feel as if they are inadequate as mothers and do not love their babies as much as the breastfeeding mothers do. Babies need to be loved, kissed, held, and touched for their emotional health, physical well-being, and happiness. At birth, this early bonding between a mother and a child is critical in molding relationships and has nothing to do with how a mother feeds her baby.

In the hospital, mothers are educated on breastfeeding following a world-wide program of the World Health Organization (WHO) and the United Nations Children's Fund (UNICEF) called the Baby-Friendly Hospital Initiative (BHFI). This initiative promotes and supports breastfeeding and improves the care of pregnant women, mothers, and newborns. It provides maternity services in hospitals and health care facilities following the International Code of Marketing of Breast-Milk Substitutes. This code supports breastfeeding by preventing the promotion, selling, distrusting, or advertising of breast milk substitutes, such as formula and baby food.

I want to review the ten steps that hospitals and health care facilities must follow to receive the Baby Friendly® designation. My comments are in the paragraph that comes immediately after the policies.

1. Have a written breastfeeding policy promoting the benefits of breastfeeding versus formula. The promotion of these policies involves all healthcare staff of nurses, physicians, lactation consultants, and administration.

Yes, the hospitals and health care facilities that are Baby-Friendly follow the required breastfeeding policies of Baby-Friendly. Are the breastfeeding policies of Baby-Friendly beneficial for the mother and her baby?

2. All health care staff is trained. Required courses and classes on breastfeeding are required for all hospital staff caring for new mothers and babies.

I agree with the Baby-Friendly policy for educating hospital staff, but until the hospitals increase the number of lactation consultants' mothers will not adequately be assisted with breastfeeding. The staffing of lactation consultants in the hospital is low, resulting in mothers receiving brief visits, little assistance, education, or guidance concerning breastfeeding. Additionally, due to inadequate staffing of lactation consultants in the hospital, nurses must take breastfeeding courses to assist mothers. Ob-gyn nurses in doctor's offices are not mandated to take continuing education courses on breastfeeding. Many ob-gyn offices do not have lactation consultants since it is not a requirement. I wonder who helps the mothers with breastfeeding in the ob-gyn offices. In hospitals and ob-gyn offices, there is little, if any, breastfeeding educational material available to mothers. According to the Baby-Friendly Hospital Initiative, wall art of the universal sign for breastfeeding should be posted in hospitals and in ob-gyn offices to promote breastfeeding. I visited multiple ob-gyn offices, and I did not see any display of the universal sign promoting breastfeeding.

3. Inform all pregnant women about the benefits of breastfeeding.

Yes, breastfeeding classes are offered in the hospital and provide information on the benefits of breastfeeding. Multiple mothers informed me hospital provided breastfeeding classes they attended are focused on the risks of using bottles, pacifiers, and formula.

4. Initiate breastfeeding during the first hour after birth.

After your baby is born, he is placed on your chest skin-to-skin, which helps the baby adjust to his new world. Will your baby latch onto your breasts in the first hour after birth? It would be great if we lived in a perfect world and your baby did latch onto your breast in the first hour after birth, but this is not normal. The first hour after delivery, you are exhausted, in pain, and your baby is sleepy.

5. Show breastfeeding mothers how to breastfeed and maintain lactation when separated from the baby.

Mothers that have had babies in neonatal intensive care (NICU) have informed me that the lactation consultants were called for assistance with breastfeeding but never came or arrived and briefly assisted them with latching their baby. These moms stated they went home frustrated and struggled with latching their baby onto their breasts; due to inadequate assistance and guidance on breastfeeding.

6. Give infants no food or drink other than breast milk unless medically indicated.

If your baby is not latching effectively onto your breasts, fussy, and showing hunger cues, such as hand-mouth activity or playing with his tongue, he is hungry and needs feeding. It should be the mother's choice if she wants to give her baby formula. I feel it is crazy that a baby has to have a medical condition to receive formula.

7. Allow rooming-in where the baby is in the room with the mother 24 hours a day.

The reality is hospitals have a baby nursery, but mothers are not encouraged to send their baby to the nursery to rest. All mothers, breastfeeding or bottle-feeding, will feel exhausted and overwhelmed without adequate rest. I do not understand why a nurse in the hospital cannot bring the baby from the nursery to the mom, breastfeeding or bottle-feeding, when the baby shows feeding or hunger cues. Allowing mothers to send their babies to the nursery will help them rest, both mentally and physically.

8. Breastfeeding on demand.

Precisely what does "on-demand" mean? Does it mean you feed your baby whenever he wakes up, maybe every 4-5 hours? Sleepiness is normal in newborns; your baby will not receive adequate milk if he is feeding only every 4-5 hours. It is important to breastfeed your baby with every feeding cue, such as opening his eyes, hand-mouth activity, or every 2-3 hours from the day of delivery.

9. No artificial teats or pacifiers.

American Academy of Pediatrics (AAP): We do not endorse a complete ban on pacifiers, nor do we support an approach that induces parental guilt concerning their choice to use pacifiers. Five meta-analyses have shown an association between pacifier use and reduced risk of sudden infant death syndrome (SIDS). The AAP Task Force recommends pacifier use at naptime and bedtime as a SIDS-reduction strategy after breastfeeding is firmly established.

I do not know if you are aware, but sucking is a natural need for babies. Sucking on a pacifier is called non-nutritive sucking, sucking without receiving food. This non-nutritive sucking causes endorphins, a hormone from your baby's brain, to be released. Endorphins cause your baby to feel relaxed and aid him to sleep. A pacifier should not be given in the place of feeding; if your baby is showing feeding cues, such as fussiness or hand-mouth activity, you need to feed your baby. After the baby is fed, offer a pacifier to your baby for relaxation and sleep.

10. Foster breastfeeding support upon discharge.

I find it horrible that mothers have to pay for breastfeeding assistance and education after discharge from the hospital; some hospitals offer one free visit. It depends on each mother's insurance policy if a lactation consultant visit is covered under her benefits. Multiple mothers and babies go home, and their baby has never latched. After discharge from the hospital, mothers are frustrated, scared, and struggling with their baby latching onto their breasts;

due to inadequate assistance and education. A large percentage of mothers told me that when they delivered on weekends, a holiday, or after 4 p.m., there were no lactation consultants available to help them with breastfeeding. I am sure the availability of lactation consultants varies from hospital to hospital.

Hospitals and health care facilities that receive the Baby Friendly® designation follow the protocols of the Academy of Breastfeeding Medicine (ABM). These protocols ensure a healthy newborn that is breastfeeding receives adequate energy and nutrients for his brain and other organs; supplementation is unnecessary and can be harmful in a mother establishing breastfeeding. Let's review the protocols of the ABM. My comments are in the paragraph that comes immediately after the protocols.

Clinical Protocol #1: Baby with low blood sugar (Hypoglycemia)

The protocol for the treatment of low blood sugar is to continue breastfeeding every 1-2 hours or syringe or cup feed baby 1.5 ccs of expressed breast milk, pasteurized donor human milk, or formula. If the baby's blood sugar level remains low, the baby will receive intravenous fluid (IV) with glucose (sugar) to increase his blood sugar level. Supplementation with formula is not fed to a baby to treat low blood sugar, which may interfere with the establishment of breastfeeding.[1]

According to this protocol, supplementation is not recommended after a baby breastfeeds unless a baby's blood sugar is below a certain level. In this situation, the baby is given 1.5 ccs of expressed breast milk, pasteurized donor human milk, or formula per syringe or cup. Every baby is different, and this amount of 1.5ccs of a supplement may be enough for your baby. If your baby is fussy and showing hunger cues, he should be fed an increased amount of supplemental feeding. According to this protocol, your baby would be given an IV of sugar instead of providing him expressed breast milk, pasteurized

---

1   Wright, Nancy and Kathleen Marinelli and The American Academy of Breastfeeding Medicine ABA Clinical Protocol # 1: Guidelines for Blood Sugar Monitoring and Treatment of Hypoglycemia in Term and late Preterm Neonates Revised 2014 Volume 9 November 4, 2014

donor human milk, or formula. I cannot understand denying food to a hungry baby. As health care providers, our priority is the health and comfort of the babies in our care. Mothers need to know how to recognize their baby may have low blood sugar. Some of the signs that your baby may have low blood sugar and you need to call your pediatrician are increased sleepiness, poor sucking, refusing to feed, irritability, or a high-pitched cry.

Clinical Protocol #2: This protocol concerns the initiation of breastfeeding in the hospital to begin within 30-60 minutes of life; the frequency of breastfeeding should be on-demand, and the baby should breastfeed 10-12 times in 24 hours.

After delivery, in my experience as a labor and delivery nurse and a lactation consultant, newborns are sleepy, and the mother is exhausted and in pain. I agree that after your baby is born, he should be skin-to-skin as much as possible to increase his security on the breast. The mother should observe her baby for feeding cues in the hospital, opening his eyes or hand-mouth activity. If her baby is not latching onto the breast every 2-3 hours, the mother needs to call the lactation consultant for assistance. Please take advantage of their help with latching your baby in the hospital.

Clinical Protocol #3: In this protocol, supplementation with formula is not given to a healthy, full-term newborn if he has had less than 8-12 feedings in the first 24-48 hours after birth, the newborn has lost less than 7 % of his birth weight, and the baby has no signs of illness. Included in this protocol, supplementation with formula is not given to a baby if the mother is tired, the baby is fussy, or the baby is cluster feeding.

If your baby has breastfed less than 8 to 12 feedings in 24-48 hours since birth, is fussy, and is showing hunger cues then your baby is hungry and needs supplementation with formula.. If a mother is tired and requests her baby to be given a bottle of formula so she can rest, then this should be the mother's choice. A sleepy baby that is breastfeeding poorly needs supplementation with formula. A baby breastfeeding frequently for brief periods needs supplementation with formula, which indicates an inadequate breast milk supply. *The definition of cluster feeding is when your baby is breastfeeding frequency with short periods of feeding. When a baby is cluster feeding, he is hungry and needs supplementation with formula. The decision of when and if formulas are given to a baby should be the mother's choice, not according to protocols.*

Testimonials from Mother

- "The lactation consultant in the hospital came into my room and briefly observed me breastfeeding; she never came back."
- "No one in the hospital helped me with breastfeeding."
- "I delivered my baby by cesarean section. I was not allowed to send my baby to the nursery so that I could get rest."
- "I had to sign a consent form to feed my baby formula as if it was poison."
- "I was instructed to hand express my breast milk, but I only had drops of milk. My baby was so hungry. I had to beg the nurses for formula."

Every mother and baby are different. We need to teach and guide each mother on breastfeeding techniques as individuals, instead of following protocols and policies. Adequate nutrition for baby is most important. From the day of conception, mothers are advised on breastfeeding and overwhelmed with information on the rights and wrongs of every aspect of feeding their newborns. Mothers feel pressured to breastfeed, are fearful of using a bottle, and are scared to use formula. If a mother does not have an adequate breast milk supply, the baby will need supplementation using a formula as her baby's food source. Moms may feel that they are harming their baby's health if they feed their baby formula. More than one million babies are given formula every day for their nutrition. If formulas were as risky as portrayed, then these children would be ill or dead. A documented risk concerning the use of formula as a baby's food source is the possibility that formula can alter the bowel (intestinal) flora, increasing the chance of a baby having an intestinal infection or diarrhea. We would currently have millions of sick babies with intestinal disorders and severe diarrhea if this were true. There are multiple reasons a baby may need formula, such as medical conditions of mom or baby, mother having a low breast milk supply, prematurity, your baby is dehydrated, jaundice, or has an inadequate weight gain.

I want to discuss breastfeeding policies from the Academy of Breastfeeding Medicine (ABM) and the American Academy of Pediatrics (AAP) concerning babies receiving supplements of formula and the support and respect of mothers who chose to give their baby formula. My comments are in the paragraph that comes immediately after the policies.

1. A breastfeeding policy from ABM concerns hospitals requiring a doctor to write an order for a baby to receive supplements of formula when medically needed for a baby and a signed consent from the mother for a baby to receive supplements of formula when it is not medically indicated

Why should a doctor's order and signed consent from the mother be needed for her baby to receive formula as her baby's food source? The reason is: the ABM suggests feeding a baby formula may be an unnecessary risk to the baby's health. I am confused. Why is it not an unnecessary risk for a baby to receive formula in NICU to save a baby's life, for an adoptive mom to give formula to her baby, or for babies to receive formula in cases of medical conditions of the mother or the baby? As per the ABM policy, if a mother chooses to bottle- feed her baby formula, it is considered an unnecessary risk to the baby's health; but using a formula as a baby's food source as mentioned in the above circumstances, is not considered an unnecessary risk to the baby's health. Does this breastfeeding policy contradict feeding a baby formula as his food source an unnecessary risk to the baby's health only if a mother chooses to use formula?

2. A breastfeeding policy for newborns from the AAP concerns treating mothers who choose not to breastfeed for medical or personal reasons with respect and support.

- *Are mothers who chose to bottle-feed their baby with formula treated with respect and support when hospitals place signs on the breastfeeding mothers' cribs stating, "My Mother Loves Me, She is Breastfeeding"?*

- *Are bottle-feeding mothers treated with respect and support when a doctor's order and signed consent from the mother is needed to receive formula for her baby in the hospital?*

- *I read an article, published in The Washington Post in September 2014, concerning a mother's decision to bottle–feed. The article, "As hospitals go 'baby-friendly,' some mothers feel slighted," discusses a mother who stated she had informed the labor and delivery nurse she decided not to breastfeed due to traveling. The Mother said, "Yet right after my daughter was born, they were ripping open my gown and trying to set up my baby to breastfeed. It was uncomfortable." In my opinion, this mother was not given the respect or support of her decision to bottle- feed with formula.[2]*

- *In a personal story, a mother of twins told me she was at her pediatricians' office, and her babies began to cry. She realized she forgot their bottles of formula. She asked the office staff for formula and was told, "We do not offer formula anymore; we are baby-friendly." When a pediatricians' office does not supply formula for bottle-feeding mothers, is this supportive?*

These are a few examples where bottle-feeding mothers were not treated with respect and support, and the policies from ABM and the AAP were not implemented.

---

2 Schulpe, Brigid: Article : As Hospitals Go Baby Friendly, Some Mothers Feel Slighted , Washington Post September 2014

As I read these protocols and policies, the main focus is on the mother's bottle-feeding their baby formula and taking risks with their baby's health. Why? Infant formula is a food providing nutrition for infants and babies less than 12 months of age. Formula manufacturers are required to register with the Food and Drug Administration (FDA). "FDA sets high-quality standards for the safety and nutritional quality of infant formulas during this critical time of development," says Stephen Ostroff, M.D., FDA's acting chief scientist. The FDA conducts yearly inspections of all facilities that manufacture infant formula. All formula is approved, tested, and meets all requirements of the FDA.

We know no formula can ever take the place of breast milk. I think it is essential to discuss the ingredients of infant formula: water, proteins, fats, vitamins, minerals, and carbohydrates. Infant formulas also contain probiotics called friendly bacteria. Probiotics can help suppress organisms' growth, help support the baby's digestion, and increase the baby's immune system. I want to review the essential nutrients in formulas approved for the growth and development of babies.

- DHA: (Docosahexaenoic acid) is an omega-3 fatty acid essential for developing your baby's nervous system, brain, and eyes. It also increases your baby's immune system.

- ARA: (Arachidonic acid) is an omega-6 unsaturated fatty acid that helps develop your baby's brain and eyes.

- Vitamin E: Protects the developing cells in your baby's body

- Lutein: Promotes the development of your baby's eyes and brain.

- Vitamin D: Increases the strength in your baby's bones by increasing the absorption of iron.

- Iron: Aids in your baby's motor development and brain development.

- Choline: Promotes your baby's brain development.

- Nucleotides: Supports the development of your baby's immune and digestive system.

As we can see, formula is not breast milk. Formulas are nutritional food for your baby tested and approved to ensure that these products are safe and support healthy growth in infants who consume them.

A Breastfeeding Nightmare Story: I worked with a nurse who told me her nightmare; concerning the Baby-Friendly protocols in the hospital where her grandchild was born.

"My daughter thought breastfeeding was going well, according to the brief observation in the hospital by the lactation consultant. At the 2-week weight check, my granddaughter had lost more than 15 % of her birth weight, and she was dehydrated and jaundiced. My grandchild was admitted to the hospital and placed on a blanket for jaundice. My daughter was told, per the nurses and the doctors, the hospital was' Baby-Friendly,' and my granddaughter would not receive any food source other than breast milk; unless medically indicated. My daughter was instructed to continue to breastfeed and pump for 24 hours. After 24 hours of breastfeeding, my grandchild was still dehydrated with dry, cracked lips. The nurse informed my daughter, intravenous fluid (IV) would be given to my granddaughter for hydration. I did not understand why my granddaughter would need an IV when she could suck and swallow, but feeding my grandchild formula was denied. After 24 hours of IV hydration, my grandchild had not improved, and formula was given. My granddaughter became more alert, had increased amounts of wet and bowel movements, and her lips were no longer dry and cracked. My daughter and grandchild were discharged from the hospital. My daughter continued to breastfeed successfully."

Mothers are informed and directed per protocols and policies of the AAP and ABM on how to breastfeed, when to breastfeed, how many times a day to breastfeed, reasons not to supplement, and avoidance of bottles and pacifiers. Mothers are overloaded with restrictions about breastfeeding. We wonder why moms are so fearful and nervous concerning feeding their babies. All mothers, breastfeeding or bottle-feeding, should observe their baby for feeding cues instead of following directions from protocols. I agree with the policies of 'Baby-Friendly' on the importance of educating mothers, increasing their knowledge, decreasing their fears, and increasing their confidence in breastfeeding. In my experience, multiple mothers have described breastfeeding classes they have attended as being focused on the risks of formula and the increased risk of SIDS with bottle-feeding with formula. Can you imagine the guilt a mother would feel if she fed her baby a bottle of formula and her baby died of SIDS?

What is SIDS? Sudden infant death syndrome (SIDS) is the unexpected death of an infant. SIDS is the leading category of non-accidental deaths between one month and one year of age. SIDS affects one in 3000 babies in the UK and one in 2000 babies in the US.

Studies have revealed that the reasons for SIDS are thought to be smoking in the household, co-sleeping of mom and her baby, a baby sleeping on his stomach, over-heating, mother drinking alcoholic beverages, mother using illegal drugs, prematurity, and a baby sleeping on soft surfaces; such as pillows, blankets, or a waterbed. Bottle-Feeding is not listed as a reason for SIDS, as stated in an article in the British Medical Journal (BMJ), Bottle Feeding, and the Sudden Infant Death Syndrome.[3][4]

---

3   Article: Boston Children's Hospital SIDS, Symptoms and Causes 2012

4   Bottle feeding and the Sudden Infant Death Syndrome *BMJ* 1995; 310 doe: https://doi. org/10.1136/bmj.310.6972.88 (Published 14 January 1995) Cite this as: BMJ 1995; 310

I understand why mothers are fearful of breastfeeding. To decrease breastfeeding mothers' fear, they can use their senses of sight and hearing to determine if their baby is hungry, tired, or uncomfortable. Most importantly, moms need to relax and enjoy their baby, breastfeeding or bottle-feeding.

Breastfeeding is not mandatory; it is a choice of feeding method. All mothers need respect and support of their choice to breastfeed or bottle-feed. In the next chapter, we will discuss the benefits of breastfeeding for mom and baby if a mother chooses to breastfeed.

Chapter 2:

Benefits of Breastfeeding and Reasons Mothers Cannot Breastfeed

According to Dr. Ruth Lawrence, "Breastfeeding is hydration, nutrition, and protection against disease and infection. It is comfort, warmth, and security, as well as breastfeeding, which is more than just milk. It is the best nutrition possible for the human infant and child. The process creates a human bond between mother and infant. An added bonus is the collection of benefits for the mother that lasts a lifetime."

You would be surprised how many women do not realize the benefits of breastfeeding. Let's discuss breastfeeding benefits for both mom and baby.

There are multiple breastfeeding benefits for your baby. Believe it or not, breast milk will save you money, it is free, it is the perfect instant meal for your baby, and it continually changes to meet your baby's growing needs. When you breastfeed, your baby receives his first vaccination, which contains antibodies and increases his immune system. Breastfed babies have a lower risk of developing eczema, allergies, asthma, diabetes, cancer, and obesity. Breast milk is easily digested and stimulates the growth of friendly bacteria called probiotics; this friendly bacterium lines the baby's intestines, preventing diarrhea, constipation, and infections. Breastfed babies have an increase in their IQ scores and have improved vision and hearing. A breastfeeding baby sucks differently from a bottle-feeding baby; this aids in developing the baby's teeth and jaw.

Breastfeeding has multiple benefits for the mother, as well. Breastfeeding is the perfect time to relax and bond with your baby. This relaxing, calming feeling is caused by a release of brain hormones called prolactin and oxytocin. Prolactin is produced from stimulation to the breast by your baby breastfeeding or pumping your breasts. Oxytocin is released when the baby licks or latches onto your breast, causing your uterus to contract. The contraction of your uterus causes your uterus to return to pre-pregnant size, the size of your fist. After your baby is delivered, the placenta, an organ attached to the uterine wall and exchanges nutrients and wastes to and from mom and baby via the mothers' umbilical cord, detaches from the uterine wall causing bleeding. The contraction of your uterus, resulting from baby licking or latching onto your breasts, causes the release of oxytocin, which decreases bleeding. Another advantage of breastfeeding is weight loss caused by the increase in metabolism or an increase in calories' burning. Mothers have a lower risk of developing cancers, high blood pressure, osteoporosis, and diabetes.

There are multiple advantages to breastfeeding for both mother and baby. We have to be realistic; there are times when a mother cannot breastfeed or totally breastfeed for numerous reasons. Let's discuss some of these reasons.

When a mother has insufficient or under-developed milk-producing glands in her breast, she may have a decrease in her milk supply. This improper development of the milk ducts and the glandular tissue is called hypo-plastic breasts; it is caused by abnormal hormone levels estrogen and progesterone. Estrogen is responsible for the growth of the milk ducts, and progesterone controls the development of the glandular tissue. Mothers with hypo-plastic breasts should consult with a lactation consultant to discuss the possible need to increase pumping and the possible need to supplement her baby with formula from inadequate milk production. It is okay to supplement your baby with formula, providing him with needed nutrition. Mothers should not feel bad or guilty for not being able to breast-feed fully. It is essential these mothers continue to be followed by a lactation consultant to monitor the baby's weight, monitor the baby's output of wet and bowel movements, and monitor the mother's milk production.

Some mothers taking medications for physical or psychological problems are not approved for breastfeeding. Mothers using drugs, such as cocaine, heroin, opioids, or any street drugs, should not breastfeed. We know that these drugs will go directly to the baby by the umbilical cord during pregnancy and transmitted to the baby by breast milk.

Human Immunodeficiency Virus (HIV)-positive mothers are advised not to breastfeed. HIV is a virus that attacks the immune system and is spread through blood, other body fluids, and breast milk. A mother who has herpes simplex, with lesions present on the breast, is encouraged not to breastfeed.

Breast surgery can possibly affect milk production. It is essential to inform your ob-gyn and lactation consultant of any breast surgery. Mothers who have had breast surgery should be followed by a lactation consultant to monitor the baby's weight, monitor the baby's output of wet and bowel movements, and monitor the mother's milk production. Augmentation (implants) usually does not interfere with milk production, but breast reduction may possibly affect nerves and milk ducts, affecting milk supply. I recommend mothers who have had breast surgery begin pumping their breasts on the day of delivery for 10-15 minutes after each feeding with every feeding cue of their baby, such as opening his eyes, hand-mouth activity, or every 2-3 hours.

There are times when mothers deliver their babies early; these babies are considered premature. It depends upon how many weeks premature your baby was born; in certain situations, premature babies are given formula containing higher calories, protein, and vitamins. When a mother delivers a preterm baby, she is under stress from being separated from her baby in NICU. She is worried about her premature baby. These mothers produce stress hormones called cortisol, which affects milk production. Mothers who deliver their babies before 37 weeks may have decreased milk production from immature mammary development. It is important mothers who deliver prematurely begin pumping their breasts on the day of delivery for 15-20 minutes every 2-3 hours day and night with a hospital grade breast pump.

Some mothers have a condition called galactosemia, a genetic disorder that prevents the digestion of galactose or lactose, a milk sugar found in breast milk, dairy products, and specific formulas. Galactosemia causes sugars to build up in the bloodstream of the baby, causing damage to internal organs. These mothers are advised not to breastfeed. This genetic disease is included in the mandatory newborn screening before mom and baby are discharged from the hospital.[5]

As you can see, there are multiple reasons a mother cannot breastfeed or cannot totally breastfeed. In these situations, their baby may need to be given formula for adequate nutrition. We know that no formula can ever take the place of breast milk. The formula companies state in their pamphlets and advertisements that they do not want their formula to take the place of breast milk. Multiple mothers say they feel guilty using formulas; information received from hospital breastfeeding class that formula is harmful to their baby's health. What is the meaning of guilt, a fact of wrongdoing? A mother is not doing anything wrong if she chooses to bottle- feed her baby formula. I have had multiple mothers ask me, "Can I give my sore nipples a break from nursing? They are cracked, bleeding, and are so painful. I feel so guilty if I give my baby a bottle of formula." These feelings of guilt are from information given to a mother before pregnancy, during pregnancy, and after delivery. Mothers need to be offered emotional

---

5   Lawrence Ruth A. Article A Review of the Medical Benefits and the Contraindications to Breastfeed in the United Sates. Maternal and Child Health Bulletin, Arlington, VA, 1997 (is not copyrighted and free duplication)

support and validation of their feelings. A mother with sore, cracked nipples needs assistance, guidance, and a treatment plan. Included in this treatment plan, I would advise this mother with sore, cracked nipples to stop breastfeeding for 12-24 hours, bottle-feed with formula or pumped milk with every feeding cue of her baby or every 2-3 hours, and pump her breasts on low for 10-15 minutes after bottle- feeding. In my experience, after 12-24 hours of resting her nipples, the mother is breastfeeding with no pain, and mother and baby are happy. Why should a mother suffer from painful breastfeeding when she can treat her nipples, rest her nipples, supplement, pump, and continue breastfeeding after her nipples are healed?

"No family should ever feel guilty or ashamed for formula feeding," says Dr. Steven Abrams.

In an op-ed for *The Washington Post*, three psychiatrists wrote: " that although the benefits of breastfeeding are backed by science, the recommendations carry the force of a threat: If I don't breastfeed, my child is more likely to get sick; if I don't breastfeed, my child won't be as smart; if I don't breastfeed, *I'm not a good mother.*" Here's what not enough people talk about: "Just as new babies are vulnerable, so are their mothers. And a mother's mental health is crucial not just to her but also to her baby. A depressed and anxious mother cannot provide the nurturing that her baby needs to develop and grow. And if that depression and anxiety are caused or worsened by the breastfeeding experience, breastfeeding isn't worth it."

Personal story: I assisted a mother who had a firm opinion of formula. Her baby was admitted to the hospital for failure to thrive, inappropriate weight gain for the baby's age. The mother was directed to come to me for assistance with breastfeeding for low weight gain. I was amazed when I saw the baby; he was six weeks old and weighed 7 pounds. His ribs were showing, and he was very pale and fragile. I asked the mother if she was supplementing her baby with formula. She stated, "Formula is bad for my baby. I am breastfeeding on demand, around every 3 hours."

Mother verbalized that she was given these instructions in the hospital. I assisted the mother with positioning and latch-on. The baby latched onto her breasts for 2-3 minutes, then fell asleep. I evaluated her breast milk production. I hand expressed very little milk. I asked the mother if she had been pumping. She stated, "I do not like pumping; I only want to breastfeed." My evaluation of this mother was an inadequate stimulation to her breast from the baby or breast pump, an insufficient milk supply, and her baby receiving a low intake of breast milk; this resulted in her baby's inadequate weight gain for his age. Before this appointment, the baby was evaluated in the hospital for low weight gain with barium tests and blood tests; and the results were all normal. This baby could suck and swallow without any difficulties. My question: if her baby could suck and swallow, why was formula not given to this baby in the hospital for an inadequate weight gain? Why did this baby have to be admitted to the hospital, have a barium exam, and blood work? The reason is that this mother feared formula and pumping. I recommended that the mother breastfeed and supplement with formula every 2-3 hours or per her baby's feeding cues. I advised her to only breastfeed for 5-7 minutes on each breast due to low milk supply. I instructed her to supplement her baby with formula after breastfeeding and pump her breasts 15-20 minutes after each feeding to increase her milk supply. I scheduled the mother a follow-up appointment in 7-10 days to evaluate the baby's weight and the mother's milk supply. At the follow-up appointment, the baby's weight and the mother's milk supply was increasing.

Formulas are an approved supplementation for a baby's nutrition. We know formula is not breast milk; formula is an option for mothers to feed their babies. There can be multiple reasons formulas are vital to a baby's health. For instance, mom or baby may have an illness, medications not approved for breastfeeding, maternal surgery, prematurity, and low milk supply. A formula is necessary when a baby has a greater than 10

% weight loss after birth or has a low weight gain. We need to live in the real world, not an imaginary world. Mothers feel pressured to breastfeed before and after conception. I think breastfeeding provides many benefits to moms and babies, but breastfeeding is not for every mom. Mothers should never feel guilty if they do not want to breastfeed. Breastfeeding is a choice, not a right or wrong. All mothers want to love and bond with their babies, whether breastfeeding or bottle-feeding. It is unfortunate when I hear moms say they cannot bond with their babies unless they breastfeed; this information is learned. What is the definition of bonding; a close emotional tie between people, such as establishing a relationship between a mother and her newly born infant. The definition of bonding does not include how a mother feeds her baby. A bond between a mother and baby is not affected by the feeding method. A bottle-feeding mother can bond with her baby as well as a breastfeeding mom. If the bottle-feeding mother wants skin-to-skin contact as the breastfeeding mother, she can take off her shirt and remove the baby's clothes down to his diaper.

The reality is mothers are stressed with expectations of feeding their baby, caring for themselves physically and mentally, caring for family, caring for other siblings, and going back to work 5-6 weeks after giving birth. Mothers are expected to be Super Moms; it is no wonder that many feel sad, exhausted, and frustrated. Mothers should not feel guilty if they choose to give their baby a bottle of formula or offer a pacifier to soothe their baby to sleep. We live in a democracy; we have choices. When it comes to choosing how to feed our babies, we brainwash our mothers. Mothers are informed, "Breast is Best," even before conception. Mothers are regularly told that they are not going to be good mothers unless they breastfeed. We are instilling guilty feelings by making them believe they are hurting their babies if they give formula. Moms become so obsessed that they feel they have to breastfeed, even if they do not want to. Sometimes a mom has tried her best, and for numerous reasons, breastfeeding is not successful. Multiple moms have stated that they feel like a failure when they are having a difficult time with breastfeeding or breastfeeding is not successful. Mothers tell me they read and hear breastfeeding is natural. These mothers then say, "If breastfeeding is so natural, what is wrong with me that I cannot breastfeed?" If breastfeeding is not successful, mothers become anxious and upset. In this situation, I would offer the mother multiple options. I can continue to assist the mother with breastfeeding as long as she wants; the mother can pump and give her baby pumped breast milk in a bottle or stop breastfeeding and give her baby formula via a bottle. I do not make her feel she is less of a mother; I validate her feelings; I praise her for her efforts and Respect her decision.

If a mother chooses to breastfeed, she needs to understand the importance of breast milk production. Without breast milk, a mother cannot breastfeed. In the next chapter, we will discuss how breast milk is made and how breast milk changes to meet your baby's growing needs.

Chapter 3:

Stimulation of the Breast Makes Milk

The more I assist mothers with breastfeeding, the more I realize mothers are not adequately educated on how breast milk is made and how to maintain a milk supply. I feel breastfeeding education should begin at the pre-conception visit to the doctor's office and continue throughout the pregnancy at each prenatal visit. Throughout the pregnancy, the ob-gyn should ask mothers about any medical conditions that can affect milk production. Mothers I have assisted with breastfeeding have informed me that their breasts were not evaluated for breastfeeding at their prenatal visits, nor were any medical history that could affect breastfeeding discussed.

Multiple mothers who attended a breastfeeding class verbalized the information covered was focused on the dangers of bottles, pacifiers, and formula; the production and maintenance of milk supply were briefly discussed. All new moms need to understand how milk is produced, how milk is released from the breast (let-down), and how milk is transferred from breast to baby by sucking and swallowing. Your breast, brain, and baby work together for adequate milk production, milk release, and milk transfer. Before we discuss how your breast, brain, and baby work together to make milk, we need to understand how and where breast milk is produced and stored. Your breast milk is made deep inside your breast by the mammary glands or glandular tissue.

Let's review the anatomy of the breast consisting of:

- Alveoli: Grape-like clusters of cells deep inside the breast that make and store breast milk

- Ducts: Tubes (roads) carry the milk from the alveoli to the nipple

- Areola: Brown area around the nipple, which can vary in size from mother to mother

- Nipple: Raised tissue located in the center of the areola with multiple openings that allow milk to flow out of the breast to the baby

- Montgomery glands: Tissue on the areola that looks like pimples. These secreting glands produce an oily, antibacterial substance that decreases bacteria on the nipple and areola. The oil from the glands reduces friction on the areola while the baby is nursing. Washing your breasts directly with soap will dry up the antibacterial substance from the Montgomery glands.

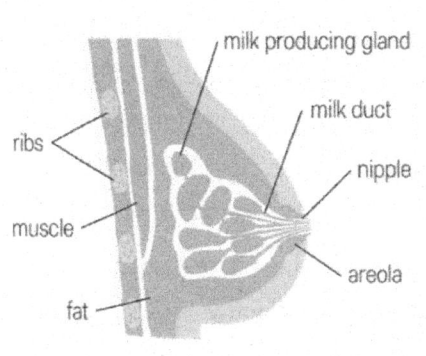

MAMMARY GLAND

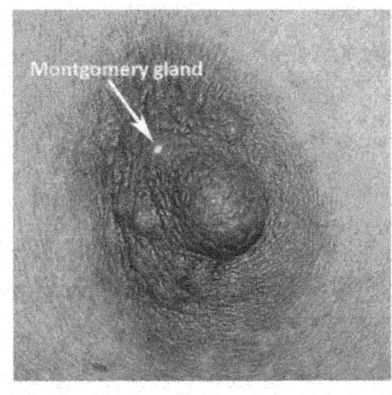

Used by permission:
Figure 19a
Nicholson B T, Harvey J A, Cohen M A. Nipple-Areolar Complex: Normal Anatomy and Benign and Malignant Processes. RadioGraphics 2009;29:509-523.

The breast's glandular tissue consists of milk-producing glands and milk ducts developed during a girls' teenage years. As we have discussed earlier, when the milk ducts and glandular tissue are not adequately developed, it is called insufficient, under-developed milk-producing glands, or hypoplastic breasts. Young women may notice that their breasts appear different; one breast may appear larger than the other breast, or her breasts may be spaced widely apart. Some women may have cone- or tubular-shaped breasts; these may or may not be hypo-plastic breasts. It is essential to discuss with your ob-gyn if you notice less than a one-cup change in your breasts' size during your pregnancy, as this can be a sign of hypo-plastic breasts. Breast milk production can be affected by hypoplastic breasts; it is vital to consult with a lactation consultant. The lactation consultant will monitor your baby's weight, monitor your baby's output of wet diapers and bowel movements, and monitor your milk production. Mothers with hypo-plastic breasts may possibly need to pump after each feeding for the duration of breastfeeding. These mothers need to be aware that even with pumping, they may not have a full breast milk supply; supplementation with formula may be necessary for the baby's adequate nutrition.

The external size of your breasts does not affect the amount of breast milk your breasts can make. The amount of fully developed glandular tissue inside your breast does make a difference in how much milk can be produced and stored. Small breasts (the container) will have a smaller amount of glandular tissue, producing and storing smaller amounts of breast milk.[6] Larger breasts have a more considerable amount of glandular tissue producing and storing more breast milk. A mother with smaller breasts may have to breastfeed more often than a woman with large breasts because of her breasts' storage capacity. The mother with smaller breasts may have to breastfeed every 2 hours; the mother with larger breasts may only need to breastfeed every 3 hours.

How is your brain involved in breast milk production? Breast milk production begins as colostrum around 16 weeks of pregnancy, which continues to a few days after delivery. Breast milk production does not progress during pregnancy due to pregnancy hormones from the placenta, estrogen, and progesterone. These hormones prevent a rise in a hormone

---

6   Mohrbacher Nancy Breastfeeding Answers Made Simple Hale Publishing, Amarillo Texas 2010 Page 399-400

from your brain called prolactin or the milk-making hormone. Without prolactin, milk production will not progress. Do not be concerned if you do not leak colostrum during your pregnancy; this is not an indicator of inadequate milk production. If you do leak drops of colostrum, wear a breast pad to keep your nipples dry.

Most mothers do not realize that milk production occurs in all women, whether they choose to breastfeed or choose not to breastfeed. Milk production begins with the delivery of your baby and the delivery of the placenta. At this time, the pregnancy hormones from the placenta, estrogen, and progesterone, are no longer needed. Your brain is then signaled, from your baby breastfeeding or pumping your breasts, causing prolactin to rise.

During breastfeeding or pumping, nerves from the nipple send messages to the mother's brain, indicating that baby needs food. These messages stimulate the mother's brain to release hormones called prolactin and oxytocin. Prolactin stimulates the alveoli deep inside the breast to make milk; it also maintains and regulates milk production. Oxytocin causes the cells surrounding the alveoli to contract and squeeze the breast milk from deep inside the breasts, through the milk ducts, out the nipple, and into the baby's mouth or pump. This process of your breast milk flowing through your milk ducts is called let-down or Milk Ejection Reflex (MER). Some mothers feel a tingling sensation in their breasts when their milk flows into their milk ducts; other mothers think nothing. Do not worry if you do not have a let-down of your milk immediately; when you are breastfeeding or pumping, your breast milk can take 1-3 minutes to flow through your milk ducts. Mothers may feel cramping from the tightening of their uterus as it returns to pre-pregnant size, caused by the release of oxytocin with breastfeeding or pumping. Prolactin and oxytocin are called the mothering hormones, increasing relaxation and feelings of love and attachment.

Your baby has the lead role in milk production. At birth and the first few weeks after birth, when your baby breastfeeds, he stimulates the mother's brain to produce prolactin receptors; located on the milk-producing cells inside of your breast. Prolactin receptors increase the production of prolactin, the milk-producing hormone, which increases milk production. Milk production at this time is hormone-driven. The more prolactin receptors produced by stimulation of the breast, breastfeeding, or pumping your breasts, the more milk mother will make. If stimulation of the breast by your baby cannot occur because the baby is ill, sleepy, or has a sucking problem, the mother must pump her breasts to keep prolactin receptors elevated, increasing prolactin levels; for continued milk production.

Your breast, brain, and baby work together for milk production. After engorgement, around 3-4 days after delivery, milk production is maintained through supply and demand. When your breasts are full of milk, less milk is made; when your breasts are empty, more milk is made. When your breasts are full of milk, your brain will release a hormone called prolactin inhibiting factor (PIF). This hormone decreases the production of prolactin, which reduces breast milk production. A mother must breastfeed or pump her breasts every 2-3 hours from the day of delivery to increase prolactin receptors, increase prolactin levels, and prevent PIF release, which results in long-term milk supply.

In the following chapter, we will discuss the transition of milk from colostrum to mature milk and multiple reasons for a delay or failure of this progression.

Chapter 4:

Transition of Breast Milk from Birth to Full Milk Production

Multiple mothers I have assisted with breastfeeding say, "My mother and sister did not make enough milk; I do not think I can breastfeed either." Please do not compare yourself to your mother, sister, or friend, who could not breastfeed. Every mother is different; if you want to breastfeed, try before saying you cannot.

The production and maintenance of milk supply is the basis of breastfeeding. When your baby is born, I do not want you to be concerned that your breasts feel soft after birth; this does not mean you will not produce milk. Your breast milk supply will slowly increase with breastfeeding or pumping. Remember, your baby has never seen a breast, felt a breast, or fed at your breast. At birth, your baby has to learn how to suck, swallow, and breathe in preparation for breastfeeding. After the delivery of your baby and the placenta, breast milk begins as drops. This small amount of breast milk makes it easier for your baby to practice sucking, swallowing, and breathing as your milk supply slowly increases.

Let's talk about how your breast milk supply increases and changes from colostrum to transitional milk to mature milk.

Colostrum is your first milk. Production of colostrum begins at 16 weeks of pregnancy and continues until around two days postpartum, after delivery. It is thick, sticky, yellow to orange in color, and provides fluids and nutrients to your baby. It is high in protein and carbohydrates, low in fat and sugar, and high in antibodies that fight bacteria and infections. Colostrum is easy to digest and functions as a lubricant that destroys bacteria. It has a laxative effect to assist the baby in removing the first thick stool called meconium. After you deliver your baby, you are producing around 1-2 teaspoons of colostrum, a minimal amount, which is appropriate for the size of your baby's stomach. On day one after birth, your baby's stomach is the size of a cherry, 5-7 ccs, or around 1-2 teaspoons. On the third day after birth, your baby's stomach is the size of a walnut, 27 ccs, or approximately 1 ounce. As your baby's stomach grows, you are slowly increasing your supply of breast milk.

Transitional milk is a combination of colostrum and mature milk, yellow to white, with a creamy appearance. Transitional milk is slowly produced around 3-4 days after birth, as your breasts begin to feel full and heavy. Mothers describe this as "My milk is coming in." Transitional milk provides an increase in sugar, fat, and calories, and a decrease in antibodies and protein. As your milk supply has increased, your baby's stomach's size has enlarged to the size of an apricot, 60 ccs, or around 2 ounces.

Mature milk is slowly produced around 5-7 days after birth with continued breastfeeding or pumping. Mature milk consists of two parts foremilk and hindmilk. Foremilk is the thin, watery milk that the baby drinks at the beginning of the feeding, like a water bottle that satisfies his thirst. Foremilk is like a salad before a meal (Lactation Education Resources, Vergie Hughes). It is high in lactose (sugar) and protein, low in fat and calories, and appears white or blue.[7] Foremilk assists in the growth of the baby's brain and provides the baby with energy. Hind milk is the thick, creamy, white milk baby drinks at the end of the feeding, baby's dessert. (Lactation

---

7   Murry , Donna RN BSN Article Name: Overview of Breastfeeding and Foremilk April 20 2020

Education Resources, Vergie Hughes). Hind milk consists of high protein, fat, and calories, like buttermilk. The baby must receive the hindmilk to be satisfied and gain weight. The size of your baby's stomach is the size of an extra-large egg, 80-150 ccs, or around 2.5-5 ounces.[8]

As we have previously discussed, transitional milk is a combination of colostrum and mature milk. Around 3-4 days after birth, when your transitional milk increases inside your milk ducts, your breasts will feel full and heavy, called engorgement. During engorgement, you will notice that your baby will stay awake longer during feeding due to increased milk production. Your baby will swallow louder and more frequently, after every 2-3 sucks, from your increase in milk supply. To decrease discomfort from excessive milk production during engorgement, pump 10-15 minutes after breastfeeding. Engorgement will resolve in around 24-48 hours. After engorgement, the production of breast milk is maintained through supply and demand. When your breasts are empty from breastfeeding or pump-ing, more milk is made; when the breasts are full of milk, less milk will be made. At this time, I recommend that you get into the habit of feeling your breasts for lumps or hardened areas after each feeding. If you feel hardened areas on your breasts, your baby did not empty your milk ducts during the feeding, and milk remains inside the milk duct; the retained milk inside of the milk duct is called plugged ducts. If the hardened milk inside the milk duct is not removed, you can develop an infection of the milk duct called mastitis, decreasing milk production. Retained milk inside the milk duct can also cause the release of prolactin inhibiting factor (PIF), which will reduce the production of prolactin, decreasing milk production. To pre-vent a decrease in milk production and prevent the possible development of mastitis, after breastfeeding, feel your breasts for any hardened areas. If a hardened area is felt on your breast, I suggest pumping your breasts 10-15 minutes after feeding. Pumping to remove the retained milk will ensure that your milk ducts are empty; for adequate milk production.

---

8   Spangler, Amy Breastfeeding A Parents' Guide 7th edition Amy's Baby Company
    Atlanta Georgia 2000 Page 34

It is important to understand breast stimulation by baby or pump is mandatory for the progression of breast milk production. Multiple reasons can cause a delay in breast milk progressing from colostrum to mature milk. Let's discuss some reasons for a delay in breast milk production.

If your baby is not latching onto your breasts or has a poor latch in the hospital, you must ask for assistance from a lactation consultant. If your baby is not latching every 2-3 hours, it is vital to pump your breasts for 10-15 for adequate breast stimulation; to prevent a delay in milk production.

Giving birth to a baby born premature, before 37 weeks gestation, can affect milk production. The ability of your premature baby to breast-feed depends on how many weeks premature your baby was born. If your baby was born after 37 weeks' gestation, he is considered to be late preterm. These babies may have weak buccal or cheeks muscles, making it harder for them to latch onto your breast. To assist your late preterm baby to latch onto your breasts, I recommend using a nipple shield; until his cheek muscles become stronger. A nipple shield is a nipple–shaped, silicone sheath that is flexible, soft, and thin. It is worn over the nipple and areola, and the tip of the nipple shield has holes to allow the breast milk to pass from the shield to your baby. I want to discuss how to apply a nipple shield: turn it inside out while placing it over your nipple, pulling the nipple deeper inside the shield. Wash the shield with soap and water and air dry after each use. To help the shield cling to the breast, you can rinse it with warm water or apply lanolin cream to the inside circumference edges. If your premature baby is not latching, the mother should begin pumping her breasts on the day of delivery for 15-20 minutes every 2-3 hours; these moms should pump day and night with a hospital grade breast pump. Breast milk is very healthy for your premature baby because it aids in fat absorption, which increases the baby's brain development. Pumping takes time and effort; be patient with yourself and proud that your baby has long-term health protection from breast milk.

A delay in breast milk production can occur in women with a high body mass index (BMI) based on height and weight. Leptin, a hormone produced from fat cells, inhibits progesterone production; progesterone is necessary for glandular tissue in breast development. I recommend that mothers with high BMI begin pumping their breasts on the day of delivery for 10-15 minutes after each feeding with every feeding cue of their baby, such as opening his eyes, hand-mouth activity, or every 2-3 hours. The stimulation of pumping your breast will increase your prolactin receptors, increase your prolactin levels; preventing a delay in milk production

The baby's mouth's anatomy can affect the baby's latching onto your breast, which can interfere with breast milk production. A tight frenulum or tongue-tie is a short string or membrane attached to the bottom or floor of the baby's mouth that prevents the baby from adequately extending his tongue, increasing breastfeeding difficulties. When your baby cannot lift and extend his tongue, it can cause your nipples to be pinched, causing nipple pain; a nipple shield can be used to decrease this nipple pinching. The ineffective latching from a tongue-tie can result in insufficient stimulation to the breast, leading to decreased milk supply. Your baby will need a referral to an ear, nose, and throat doctor (ENT) to clip the frenulum (a frenotomy). After the ENT doctor clips or cuts the tongue-tie, most babies have improved latching, preventing nipple pain and increasing breast stimulation.

We forget how difficult it is for a mother and a baby during and after a cesarean section. Mothers that have a cesarean section may have a decreased milk supply for a variety of reasons. When a baby is born by cesarean section, his lungs are not adequately squeezed at the delivery, causing secretions to remain in the baby's mouth and throat. The ob-gyn will suck the secretions from the baby's mouth and throat, possibly causing the baby to have a sore throat, delaying baby latching. Pain from the incision can cause discomfort when the mother is breastfeeding. To decrease incisional pain, I recommend using a football position. Medications needed with a cesarean section can affect breastfeeding after delivery, making both mom and baby sleepy. I advise mothers who have had a cesarean section pump their breasts starting on the day of delivery for 10-15 minutes after each feeding with every feeding cue of their baby, such as opening his eyes, hand-mouth activity, or every 2-3 hours. I do not feel you need to pump at night unless your baby is not latching; you need rest for your physical and mental health. Pumping your breasts, starting the day of delivery, increases prolactin receptors, and increases prolactin levels, preventing a delay in milk production.

There can be issues that affect milk production after the delivery of your baby. After your baby is born, the placenta is delivered. If any parts of the placenta remain inside the uterus, it can affect your milk production. The placenta produces hormones called estrogen and progesterone. Estrogen and progesterone prevent a rise in prolactin, the milk-making hormone, resulting in a delay in breast milk production. Retained parts of the placenta remaining inside the uterus can decrease blood supply to the pituitary gland, responsible for prolactin and oxytocin production, affecting milk production. Oxytocin is responsible for the let-down of your breast milk. It also causes the mother's uterus to contract after delivery, controlling bleeding; a sign of retained placenta is excessive blood loss after delivery.

As we have discussed, for breastfeeding to be successful, your breast, brain, and baby have to work together to make milk. The following chapter will discuss how a sleepy baby, inadequate breast stimulation, and insufficient prolactin production can affect milk supply. It is essential to breastfeed or pump your breasts every 2-3 hours, especially the first two weeks after birth, increasing prolactin receptors and increasing prolactin levels, resulting in good, long-term milk production.[9]

---

9   Mohrbacher, Nancy IBCLC, FaIL CA Breastfeeding Answers Made Simple. A Guide for Helping Mothers Hale Publishing, Amarillo Texas 2010 page 394

Chapter 5:

Breastfeeding Problems the First Two Weeks After Birth

I have noticed two main breastfeeding problems that can occur during the first few weeks after birth sleepy newborn and mother's milk supply.

Mothers I have assisted with breastfeeding are not aware that all newborns are exhausted from birth to day 14 or longer, they fall asleep quickly at the breast, and each baby has different degrees of sleepiness. If your baby is allowed to sleep at the breast, the results will be a decreased stimulation to the breast and a reduced milk supply. It is necessary to stimulate your sleepy newborn to stay awake and breastfeed. As your baby is breastfeeding, use your senses of hearing, seeing, and feeling to determine if your baby is falling asleep. Do you hear and see your baby swallowing during the feeding, do you see his eyes closing, and do you feel the strength of his suck decreasing? If you hear, see, or feel signs your baby is falling asleep, he needs stimulation to feed. To stimulate your baby to suck and swallow, I would like to discuss a form of breast stimulation called breast compression. Compression of the milk ducts causes a let-down of your milk into your milk ducts and stimulates your baby to swallow, keeping the baby awake to breastfeed. There are multiple advantages of breast compression, increasing the strength of your baby's suck, increasing the stimulation to your breast, and increasing milk production.

The step-by-step process of performing breast compression:

- Position one hand on your breast resembling a 'C 'shape

- Place your thumb above your breast and your fingers below your breast, not touching the areola.

- Slide your thumb down toward your nipple, stopping at the edge of the areola

- Lift thumb, and repeat

When you hear your baby swallowing, he is awake and receiving food. It can be very challenging to keep a sleepy baby awake to breastfeed for him to provide stimulation to your breasts to make breast milk. I want to discuss the steps of breastfeeding a sleepy newborn, including ways to stimulate him to stay awake. After you observe your baby demonstrating feeding cues, such as opening his eyes and hand-mouth activity, undress your baby down to the diaper. Skin-to-skin contact, also known as kangaroo care, will prevent your baby from becoming overheated, increasing sleepiness. [10]Do not be concerned that your baby is undressed, as your body heat will keep him warm. During the feeding, your baby will show you signs he is falling asleep; his eyes will be closing, and his sucking will feel weaker; break the seal of the baby's suck with your finger in the corner of his mouth and rotate your baby to the opposite breast. Before placing the baby on your opposite breast, you will need to stimulate him by rubbing his spine or blowing into his face. Every baby has different degrees of sleepiness; you may have to rotate or change breasts for a very sleepy newborn every 5-7 minutes. If your baby is less than 37 weeks gestation, you may need to rotate breasts every 3-4 minutes for needed stimulation to keep

---

10 Ferber, S.G. and R Makhoul Article Name: The effects of skin to skin contact (kangaroo care) shortly after birth on the neurobehavioral responses of the term newborn Pediatrics 2004

your baby awake. Rotating or changing your breasts during breastfeeding will increase your baby's stimulation, increase the strength of your baby's suck, increase the stimulation to your breasts; increasing milk supply.

During the feeding, continue watching your baby for signs that his stomach is full; he will not show any hunger cues, such as fussiness, hand-mouth activity, or playing with his tongue. When your baby appears to be content, re-dress him. With this stimulation, if he is still hungry, he will open his eyes and perform a hand-mouth activity, offer Dessert, placing him back on the breast that feels more-full to finish his meal. Continue to rotate your breasts when your baby shows signs of going to sleep; breastfeed until your baby is full and content When your baby's stomach is full, he will refuse to latch. You will see his lips will be closed tightly, his arms and legs will be limp; he will not be fussy and will not demonstrate feeding cues. I want you to be aware that the main goals of every newborn are snacking and sleeping. A sleepy newborn will go to sleep, even if he is not full, not filling his tummy at each feeding. If your baby shows feeding or hunger cues, such as fussiness or hand- mouth activity, feed your baby; it does not matter how long it has been since the last feeding.

It takes time and energy to provide stimulation to your sleepy baby to stay awake and breastfeed. How long does it take to stimulate and breastfeed your sleepy newborn? I know you have been instructed in breastfeeding classes to feed your baby 2 hours from the beginning of the last feeding, but is this practical? Let's discuss why you should breastfeed your baby with every feeding cue, or every 2 hours from the End of the last feeding in the day, and every 3 hours from the End of the last feeding at night. How long does it take to feed a sleepy newborn? It may take 45 minutes to 1 hour to breastfeed your sleepy newborn, between rotating your breasts and stimulating your baby to stay awake and breastfeed. If your baby began feeding at 8 a.m., and the feeding ended at 9 a.m., your baby will not be hungry at 10 a.m., which is 2 hours from the beginning of the last feeding. Baby refusing to feed causes the mother to be concerned and frustrated. I recommend feeding your baby at 11 am, 2 hours from the end of the last feeding, which ended at 9 am. Breastfeeding your baby 2 hours from the End of each feeding is more effective; the baby is hungry, the baby breast-feeds better, and the mother receives more rest. If your baby demonstrates feeding or hunger cues before 2 hours from the end of the last feeding, feed your baby. Your baby will breastfeed better when he is hungry, resulting in the baby feeding well. If your baby is not hungry and not ready to breast-feed, he will refuse to latch onto your breasts or breastfeed poorly.

Mothers are concerned that their baby will not get enough hindmilk, the milk at the end of the feeding if they rotate their breasts during the feeding. In breastfeeding classes and the hospital, mothers are taught to leave their baby on one breast for 15 minutes and feed their baby every 3 hours. Will baby receive an adequate amount of milk if you leave your baby on one breast for 15 minutes, he falls asleep after 5-7 minutes, and the next feeding is in 3 hours? We have to be practical and use your common sense, which tells us that baby will not receive an adequate amount of breast milk. I want you to think about what happens when a baby falls asleep at the breast. The mother thinks her baby is full, and she puts him down to sleep; within 30-45 minutes after breastfeeding, her baby wakes up crying in hunger. The mother is confused; her baby has just been fed. When your baby is allowed to sleep at the breast, he will not receive adequate hind-milk and too much foremilk. Baby will have green stools, fussiness, and gas from too much foremilk. When a baby does not receive a sufficient amount of hindmilk, he will be hungry and fussy. He will have inadequate weight gain, a poor output of wet and bowel movements, and possibly becoming dehydrated and developing jaundice.

Let's discuss jaundice and how you can prevent your baby from becoming jaundice. After your baby is born, it is normal for the baby's red blood cells to break down and form bilirubin, a brown, yellow sub-stance found in the bile. The main exit for bilirubin is in the stool, via bowel movements. If your baby is feeding well and having sufficient amounts of bowel movements, the bilirubin will exit the baby's body. Suppose your baby is sleeping at the breast; he is not swallowing and does not receive an adequate amount of breast milk intake, resulting in decreased bowel movements, causing an increase in his body's bilirubin level. The elevation of bilirubin in his body can cause an increase in the sleepiness of your newborn. It is essential to rotate your breasts throughout the feeding and stimulate your baby to stay awake for adequate breast milk intake. If your baby is too sleepy to feed or breastfeeding poorly, he will not receive a sufficient amount of milk from your breast; supplementation with formula may be needed to increase bowel movements, decreasing bilirubin, and decreasing the development of jaundice.

Your baby sleeping at the breast can cause multiple issues. When your baby sleeps at the breast, he is not emptying your milk ducts. The retained milk inside your ducts can cause plugged ducts and mastitis. If your baby is not swallowing after every 2-3 sucks and is allowed to sleep at the breast, the results will be decrease stimulation to the breast; decreasing milk production. It is essential to recognize that swallowing indicates your baby is drinking and receiving milk. The amount of time that your baby is on the breast is not an indicator that the baby has received an adequate amount of food (milk). Please remember stimulation is critical to keep your baby awake for your baby to suck, swallow, and receive milk, breast-feeding, or bottle–feeding.

I want to discuss how a breastfeeding mother knows her baby is drinking and receiving milk. When I assist mothers with breastfeeding, their main concern is whether their baby is receiving milk when he is breastfeeding? Breastfeeding mothers have this concern because they cannot see how much milk their baby is drinking when he is breastfeeding; they can see how much their baby is drinking when bottle-feeding. You will not directly see how much milk your baby is drinking when you are breastfeeding, but your baby will show signs that he is receiving food. The best indicator that the baby is receiving food, as he is breastfeeding, is to use your senses of seeing, hearing, and feeling.

Let's review the signs of good or adequate breast milk supply.

- During the feeding, you will See your baby is relaxed and calm; he is not fussy.

- You will See your baby's chin pause when his mouth is full of milk

- You will See and Hear your baby is swallowing after every 2-3 sucks

- You will See breast milk leaking from your opposite breast during the feeding

- You will See milk in the corners of your baby's mouth.

- You will See your baby is having an adequate output of wet diapers and bowel movements for his age

- After the feeding, you will See your baby will not be fussy; he will be content.

- You will Feel your breasts are soft after breastfeeding; an indicator baby has emptied your milk ducts and received milk

Common sense tells us that if your baby is drinking an adequate amount of breast milk, he will gain weight and be content and happy. A baby responds to milk; when your baby sucks and receives milk, he wants to suck harder. If a baby sucks and receives little milk, the baby becomes frustrated and falls asleep.

Let's review the signs of poor or inadequate breast milk supply.

- During the feeding, you will See your baby will be fussy

- You will not See or Hear your baby swallowing after every 2-3 sucks.

- You will See your baby will want to breastfeed all of the time due to low milk supply.

- You will See that your baby will have an inadequate output of wet and bowel movements for his age.
- After feeding, you will See your baby is fussy (some mom's think this is gas or colic; this is hunger)
- You will See that your baby is sleeping poorly from hunger
- You will Feel your breasts are soft from inadequate milk supply.

I want you to be aware of some warning signs to call your pediatrician and consult with a lactation consultant. Let's discuss some of these warning signs.

- Your baby is feeding poorly
- Your baby's skin and whites of his eyes appear yellow
- Your baby's eyes have a sunken appearance
- Your baby's skin and lips are dry
- Your baby is very sleepy due to low blood sugar
- Your baby is having an inadequate output of wet diapers for his age
- Baby's wet diapers have red crystals, which indicate dehydration
- Your baby has an inadequate amount of bowel movements for his age
- Your baby has black, tarry stools on day 4-5 after birth, instead of the normal-appearing bowel movements that are liquid, yellow, and have a cottage cheese-like appearance on day 4-5 after birth.

An adequate output of wet and bowel movements for a baby's age is a good indicator your baby is getting enough food (milk).

Day 1 and 2:   1-2 wet diapers   1-2 black, tarry stools (meconium)

Day 3 and 4:   3-4 wet diapers;   3-4 green-brown transitional stools

Day 4 and 5:   4-5 wet diapers;   3-6 liquid, yellow, cottage cheese-
                                        like stools

There are times when your baby will want to eat more; these are called growth spurts. You will notice your baby will eat more frequently and breastfeed longer to compensate for the baby getting bigger and needing more milk. A growth spurt occurs around every two months and lasts around 2-3 days until your milk supply has caught up with your baby's needs. The increase in breastfeeding frequency will cause an increase in breast stimulation and an increase in milk production.

A breastfeeding mother is always worried if her baby is getting enough breast milk for adequate growth. Who determines sufficient growth for a baby? The World Health Organization (WHO) developed a standard of measuring a child's growth and development based on the infant's weight, length, and head circumference called growth charts. I want to review how the growth charts are used to evaluate the adequate growth of your baby. If your baby is at 50 % for weight and 10 % for height on a growth chart, it means that one half or 50 % of healthy babies of the same age in the United States are lighter, and the other half is heavier. When your baby is at 10 % height, that means 90 % of babies in the United States are taller than your child, and 10 % are shorter.

Using a growth chart is a guide, but doctors and lactation consultants need to evaluate each baby individually. We need to consider several things; are the mom and dad small in weight and height, is baby meeting the milestones for his developmental age, has baby grown in length, and has baby's head circumference increased (brain growth). When evaluating a newborn's weight loss or gain, a critical oversight can be as simple as verifying that the follow-up weight checks are performed with the baby's clothes always on or off. Did the nurse use the same scale for every follow-up weight?

Weight loss in newborn babies is common after birth for a variety of reasons. During labor and delivery, mothers are usually given a lot of intravenous fluid. Some mothers are in labor for a long time, during which the mother and baby are receiving and retaining fluid. The birth weight of your baby will include the weight of the retained fluid from the intravenous fluid. When your baby has a weight check 3-4 days after birth, weight loss will be noted. Pediatricians prefer less than a 10 % weight loss for a baby that is 3-4 days old; a 7 % weight loss is normal for a baby that is 3-4 days old. A reason for weight loss after birth can be different for the breastfeeding and bottle-feeding baby. Formulas have more calories and account for less weight loss in the bottle feeding baby; than the breastfeeding baby who is receiving drops of colostrum until breast milk increases around 3-4 days after birth. As we have discussed, all newborns are sleepy; it is essential to feed your baby at every feeding cue, such as opening his eyes, hand-mouth activity, or every 2-3 hours. All newborns have to be stimulated to eat throughout the feeding, whether breastfed or bottle-fed.

For a breastfeeding baby to receive adequate milk, he has to latch onto your breast correctly. In the following chapter, we will discuss the steps to latch your baby onto your breast, increasing breastfeeding success.

Chapter 6:

Comfort and Security Are Key to a Successful Latch-On

I know you have heard breastfeeding is natural but is it? Breastfeeding does not come naturally to the baby or the mother. Yes, babies have instincts for breastfeeding and can smell your milk, but does your baby know how to latch himself correctly onto your breast? We need to remember your baby has never felt skin or breastfed. After delivery, if you place the baby on your chest, he will slowly crawl up toward your nipple, using your areola as a bull's eye, and bob his little head until he latches. Allowing a baby to latch by crawling up your chest will pinch your nipples and cause pain from an incorrect latch. All newborns have weak head, neck, and back muscles. Practicing latching baby onto your breast with repeated support and guidance to baby's head, neck, and back will decrease his frustration; as he slowly learns how to breastfeed. Breastfeeding is a learned skill, like driving a car or skating; patience and practice are essential to successful breastfeeding. Positioning your baby to latch onto your breast is a process, taking one step at a time. For breastfeeding to be successful, your baby has to be comfortable. I have observed that when moms align the baby's upper lip to their nipple, support the baby's head, neck, and back, and guides baby onto the breast, breastfeeding is comfortable for both mom and baby. Your baby has to feel supported and secure to adequately suck, swallow, and transfer milk from your breasts. If your baby is not comfortable and supported at the breast, he thinks he is slipping off the breast and will cry. This insecure feeling of slipping causes the baby to turn his head from side to side and rapidly move his arms and hands to hold himself onto the breast; mothers describe baby slipping off of her breasts as "My baby fights and pushes me away. He does not want to breastfeed." It is a cycle of no support to the baby's weak head, neck, and back muscles; baby slips off the breast and mother re-latching baby onto her breasts. This insecure feeling causes your baby to be frustrated and go to sleep; he wakes up 30 minutes to 1 hour crying in hunger; the mother is frustrated and crying from exhaustion.

How do you know your baby is comfortable and latched well? My class is based on observing your baby using your senses of seeing, hearing, and feeling.

Let's review the signs of a good or effective latch.

- You will not Feel nipple pain, only a mild pulling sensation of your breast tissue.

- You will See your baby's chin pause when his mouth is full of milk

- You will Hear baby swallowing after every 2-3 sucks

- You will See your baby is relaxed with his hands open.

- You will See your baby's jaw moving as he is nursing

- You will See breast milk leaking from your opposite breast

- You will See breast milk in the corners of the baby's mouth

- You will See your baby will be content and not fussy after the feeding

- You will See no change in the color or shape of your nipples after the feeding

- Your breasts will Feel soft after feeding; your milk ducts are empty

Let's review the signs of a poor or ineffective latch.

- You will Feel nipple pain
- You will not See or Hear your baby swallowing after every 2-3 sucks
- You will See your baby appearing tense with his hands in a fist
- You will not See your baby's jaw moving during the feeding
- You will See your baby's lips looking like he is sucking on a straw
- You will See your nipples appearing white or purple after the feeding
- You will See your nipples having a pinched or lipstick shape after the feeding
- You will See your baby's cheeks indenting
- You will Hear a clicking or smacking sound
- You will See your baby fussy during and after feeding.
- Your breasts will Feel firm after feeding; as a result of your milk ducts remaining full of milk from an incorrect latch.

A poor latch on the breast can cause multiple problems in breastfeeding with the mother and baby. A poor latch can cause the mother to have sore nipples, inadequate stimulation to the breasts, and insufficient milk production. If your baby is not latching correctly, your milk ducts become engorged or overfilled with milk. Unrelieved engorgement results in retained milk inside the milk ducts, leading to pain, plugged ducts, mastitis, and a decreased milk supply. When your baby continues to latch poorly on your breasts, he will be hungry and fussy, resulting in the baby having a weight loss, becoming dehydrated, and possibly developing jaundice.

What is the process of latching your baby onto your breast? Visualize putting a puzzle together, one piece at a time. When you place a puzzle together, all of the pieces fit close together, and there is no space or gap between the puzzle pieces. Latching a baby onto the breast is like putting a puzzle together, one step at a time, ending with mother and baby skin-to-skin. There is no space or gap between your body and the baby's body, like a puzzle. Following steps for latching your baby onto the breast can be your guide to practice as you are learning to breastfeed.

Quotes from mothers I have assisted:

- "Breastfeeding is so painful, but I was told it would get better the longer I breastfeed."
- "The lactation consultants in the hospital told me my baby was latching well. I kept telling them my nipples were hurting."
- "My nipples looked pinched and lipstick shaped in the hospital. I was not told this is a sign my baby was not latching correctly."

Let's discuss the key points for positioning and latching your baby onto your breast. As a lactation consultant, I have heard so many times, "I was told to latch my baby, but I do not know how." My goal is to teach you how to latch your baby onto your breast using multiple breastfeeding positions and understanding each step. I will explain the reasons for each step of latching your baby, which will help you understand the importance of a comfortable position for both you and your baby. When mom and baby are comfortable during breastfeeding, the feeding will be enjoyable for both.

Read and review each key point of latching your baby onto your breast. Practice using a baby doll; then follow the steps for latching your baby onto your breasts.

- Skin-to-Skin/Kangaroo Care: Before breastfeeding, remove your shirt and bra and undress your baby down to his diaper.

Skin-to-skin contact with mom and baby has been proven to keep baby warm and increase bonding, breastfeeding, or bottle-feeding

- Comfortable Position: When mom and baby are comfortable, breastfeeding is more successful. To promote comfort while breastfeeding, relax in a chair or couch with your shoulders relaxed. When you position your baby to latch, always bring the baby to your breast, not breast to the baby; and bring the baby to nipple, not nipple to the baby. This process will prevent you from having poor posture from bending and twisting your body. A footstool may be helpful to decrease back strain. A firm pillow can be used to provide comfort and support for the mother and the baby. When you are positioning the pillow, adjust it slightly below the level of your nipples. Remember, your baby has never breastfed and needs assistance, support, and guidance. To assist your baby onto the pillow, place one of your hands on your baby's buttock and your opposite hand at the base of your baby's head and neck; slowly position your baby on a firm pillow such as a My Breast Friend pillow. A firm pillow will help you maintain good posture during breastfeeding, which will decrease back, shoulder, and neck pain. A pillow will also help you keep your baby skin-to-skin, decreasing the space or gap between your body and your baby's body. Throughout the feeding, your baby's head and body will remain on the pillow at all times. I want to explain each step of positioning your baby onto your breast in a comfortable position.

- I want you to perform an exercise: turn your head to the side and try to swallow; it is hard. When your baby is on his back and turns his head to the side to breastfeed, it is hard for him to swallow. It is essential to align your baby's ear, shoulder, and hip in a straight line, allowing the baby to suck and swallow in a comfortable position.

- As we have discussed, positioning your baby onto the breasts is like putting a puzzle together; the pieces are close and tight. You need to position your baby close and tight to your body by placing one of your hands on your baby's buttock and your opposite hand at the base of your baby's head and neck, sliding the baby's body towards your body until your chest and baby's chest is touching.

- It is essential to align your baby's upper lip to your nipple's to prevent nipple pain. Every mother's breasts, nipples, and areolas are different; you need to ask yourself: *Where is my nipple?* A woman with small breasts may have her nipple located in the center of her breast, while a woman with large breasts may have her nipple located low and angled down. Some nipples are angled to the right, left, up, or down; all are normal. Wherever your nipple is located is where you align your baby's upper lip. If nipple pain continues, practice aligning the baby's nose to your nipple. Every mother and baby are different; trial and error is the key to success with no nipple pain,

- We need to remember all newborns have a weak head, neck, and back, so you must provide support to your baby's head, neck, and back while breastfeeding your baby. A baby's head is like a bobblehead, and without the support, he becomes upset and cries. Providing support to your baby's head, neck, and back is essential. The web of your hand between your fingers and your thumb supports the base of your baby's neck. Your fingers are close and tight and support the baby's chin and cheeks without squeezing. Your forearm is supporting the baby along his spine.

- With the web of your hand at the base of your baby's neck, angle your wrist inward towards the middle of your baby's shoulder blades. This inward position of your wrist prevents pinching of your nipple, resulting in nipple pain. When you angle your wrist inwards, your baby's chin will be touching your areola, and your baby's nose will be pointed up. This position allows the baby to breathe and swallow easier. I want you to do another exercise: bend your head forward and try to swallow; it is hard. Baby feels the same compression to his throat if you push your baby's head down towards his chest. Avoid bending your wrist outwards, away from your baby's body. When your wrist is angled outward baby's head is pushed forward, causing the baby's nose to be blocked by your breast tissue and compression of your baby's throat, causing the baby to have difficulty breathing and swallowing.

Before attempting to latch the baby onto your breast, look down at how your baby is positioned. Your baby's head and body are on a firm pillow. Baby's body is fitting close to your body, with no spaces or gaps between your baby's chin and your areola, between your baby's upper lip and your nipple, between your baby's chest and your chest, and between your baby's stomach and your stomach? You have formed a puzzle between your body and your baby's body. Your baby's head, neck, and back are supported by your hand, wrist, and forearm.

The secret to preventing nipple pain with latch-on is to prevent your baby from closing his mouth before he latches; his upper lip or nose should be touching your nipple before latching him onto your breast. When your baby's nose or your baby's upper lip is not touching your nipple before he latches, he closes his mouth; his mouth will be narrow, like a fish, causing nipple pinching and pain. Remember, pain means stop breastfeeding and re-position your baby onto the breasts.

As you are reading each step of positioning your baby to latch onto your breast, go slowly and take one step at a time. You may have to re-latch the baby multiple times if you feel pain. Be aware that if your baby does not feel secure, supported, and comfortable at the breast; he will turn his head from side to side and flail his arms in frustration. Guiding and supporting your baby to latch decreases stress for you and your baby.

Read and follow the step-by-step instructions on latching your baby onto your breasts in the cross-cradle, football, side-lying, and cradle position.

Cross-Cradle is the most common breastfeeding position for a newborn with a weak head, neck, and back.

Follow the steps for positioning your baby in the Cross Cradle position on the left breast.

- The mother should be in a comfortable position with her shoulders relaxed

- Your baby's head and body should be supported on a firm pillow, slightly below the level of your nipples

- Place your right hand on the baby's buttock and your left hand at the base of your baby's head and neck and turn your baby on his side with his ear, shoulder, and hip in a straight line.

- Keeping your right hand on your baby's buttock and your left hand at the base of your baby's head and neck, bring the baby's body toward your body until your chest and your baby's chest is touching, and then you align the baby's upper lip to your nipple.

- Slide your right hand and forearm from your baby's buttock up the center of the baby's spine until the web of your hand, between your thumb and your fingers, touches or locks into the base of your baby's neck. Pretending baby's lower arm is attached to your wrist and forearm, use your left hand to gently slide baby's lower arm under your breast toward your back, at the same time bringing your wrist and forearm closer to the breast.

- Spread the fingers of your right hand to support the baby along his chin and cheeks. Your thumb should be near the baby's opposite ear.

- Angle your right wrist is inward, your baby's chin is touching your areola, your baby's upper lip is touching your nipple, and your baby's nose is pointed up (sniffing position).

- Slide the fingers of your left hand under your left breast, below the areola, above the baby's lower arm. Your thumb is on top of the breast above the areola.

- With your fingers and thumb of your left hand, gently squeeze your breast tissue together as if forming a sandwich.

- Using your left hand to support your left breast, slowly and softly tickle your nipple across the baby's upper lip, do not lift the breast.

- Baby will open his mouth wide and latch onto your breast.

- As needed, bring your right arm closer to your body for a complete puzzle.

Football Position is comfortable for mothers with large breasts or mothers delivered per a cesarean section. Using the football position, the baby tends to push his feet against the back of the chair or sofa; using a pillow behind your back and sitting at the edge of the chair or sofa may prevent this from occurring.

Follow the steps for positioning your baby in the football position on the right breast

- The mother should be in a comfortable position with her shoulders relaxed

- Your baby's head and body should be supported on a firm pillow, slightly below the level of your nipples

- Place your right hand on the baby's buttock and your left hand at the base of your baby's head and neck and turn your baby on his side with his ear, shoulder, and hip in a straight line.

- Keeping your right hand on your baby's buttock and your left hand at the base of your baby's head and neck, bring the baby's body toward your body until your chest and your baby's chest is touching.

- Slide your baby along your right side until the baby's upper lip touches your nipple.

- Move your right hand and forearm from your baby's buttock up the center of the baby's spine until the web of your hand, between your thumb and your fingers, touches or locks into the base of your baby's' neck.

- Spread the fingers of your right hand to support your baby along his chin and cheeks. Your thumb should be near the baby's opposite ear.

- Angle your right wrist is inward, your baby's chin is touching your areola, your baby's upper lip is touching your nipple, and your baby's nose is pointed up (sniffing position)

- Slide the fingers of your left hand under your right breast, below the areola, and above the baby's lower arm. Your thumb is on top of the breast above the areola.

- With your fingers and thumb of your left hand, gently squeeze your breast tissue together as if forming a sandwich.

- Using your left hand to support your right breast, slowly and softly tickle your nipple across the baby's upper lip, do not lift the breast.

- Baby will open his mouth wide and latch onto your breast.

- As needed, bring your right arm closer to your body for a complete puzzle.

The **Side-Lying Position** can be advantageous, especially at night.

Follow the steps for positioning your baby in the side-lying position on the right breast

- Lie on your right side, using one to two pillows under your head to view your baby more easily.
- Turn your baby on his side with his ear, shoulder, and hip in a straight line. The baby's entire body is touching your body.
- Align the baby's upper lip to your nipple.
- Position your right arm above your baby's body.
- Slide the fingers of your left hand under your right breast below the areola. Your thumb is on top of the breast above the areola.
- Slowly and softly tickle your nipple across the baby's upper lip.
- Baby will open his mouth wide and latch onto your breast.

The **Cradle Position** is a good position for the older baby with more head control.

Follow the steps for positioning your baby in the cradle position on the left breast.

- The mother should be in a comfortable position with her shoulders relaxed
- Your baby's head and body is supported on a firm pillow, slightly below the level of your nipples
- Place your right hand on the baby's buttock and your left hand at the base of your baby's head and neck and turn your baby on his side with his ear, shoulder, and hip in a straight line.
- Keeping your right hand on your baby's buttock and your left hand at the base of your baby's head and neck, bring the baby's body toward your body until your chest and your baby's chest is touching.

- Wrap your left arm around the baby's body with your baby's head in the area of your elbow. Place your left hand on the baby's buttock, positioning your baby's buttock close to your body; resulting in the baby's nose pointed up

- Using your left arm supporting the baby, align the baby's upper lip to your nipple.

- Slide the fingers of your right hand under your left breast below the areola. Your thumb is on top of the breast above the areola.

- Angle your right wrist inward, your baby's chin is touching your areola, your baby's upper lip is touching your nipple, and your baby's nose is pointed up (sniffing position).

- With your fingers and thumb of your right hand, gently squeeze your breast tissue together as if forming a sandwich.

- Using your right hand to support your left breast, slowly and softly tickle your nipple across the baby's upper lip, do not lift your breast.

- Baby will open his mouth wide and latch onto your breast.

- As needed, bring your left arm closer to your body for a complete puzzle.

The key to your baby effectively latching onto the breast is the comfort of mom and baby with proper alignment, support, and guidance. The mother is in the control seat; the baby has no knowledge or strength to guide him onto the breast. Remember, you and your baby are learning to breastfeed together.

Mothers of multiples feel anxious and concerned that they cannot breastfeed, but it is both possible and enjoyable. Working with moms of multiples, I have noticed more success when the mother breastfeeds one twin until both babies are feeding effectively and then breastfeed twins together. I would recommend starting with the football position; as time progresses, mom can experiment with other positions. Do not allow babies to sleep at the breast. When you see your babies begin to close their eyes, and their sucking decreases and weakens, you need to rotate babies to the opposite breast. Before you rotate babies to the opposite breast, you need to break the seal of the baby's suck on your breast by placing your finger into the corner of your baby's mouth and remove him from your breast. After removing babies from your breast, you need to stimulate your babies to stay awake and feed. To stimulate your babies, you can blow into their faces or rub their feet. It is normal for twins to be very sleepy; continue to rotate breasts until babies are content and showing no feeding cues. It is essential to observe the babies and breastfeed with every feeding cue, such as opening their eyes, hand-mouth activity, or every 2-3 hours day and night. Supplementation with formula or pumped milk after breastfeeding may be needed until adequate milk production is available for both babies. To increase milk production, I recommend that mothers of twins or multiples begin pumping 10-15 minutes after each feeding with every feeding cue of their babies, such as opening their eyes, hand-mouth activity, or every 2-3 hours.

I have provided some pictures of babies in the cross-cradle, cradle, football position, and twins at the breast. I want you to notice the baby's chin is touching the areola, and the baby's nose is pointed up. These babies are comfortable and breastfed well. The twins are sleepy, which is normal. Both babies nursed well with continued stimulation to stay awake.

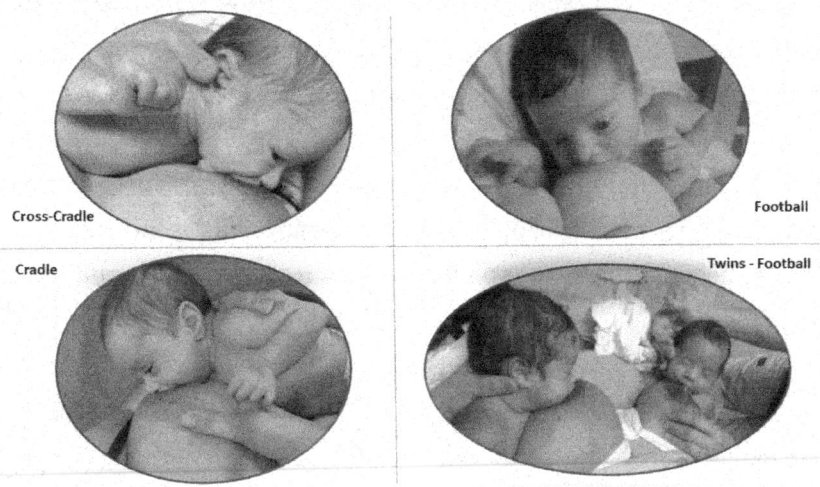

Cross-Cradle

Football

Cradle

Twins - Football

Breastfeeding should be a relaxing, enjoyable, bonding experience for you and your baby. I do not want you to be fearful of the next feeding due to frustration and pain, latching your baby onto your breasts. Remember, you are not in a race to latch your baby. You will need to take one step at a time, and it may take multiple attempts to latch your baby without pain; if pain continues, you need to call a lactation consultant for evaluation and assistance. It may take up to 3 weeks to feel comfortable breastfeeding; be patient, relax, and enjoy your baby.

Incorporating a new addition to your family is an adjustment. In time, it will feel as if your baby has always been part of your life. In the next chapter, we will discuss establishing routines and how and when to put your baby on a schedule. Establishing routines and schedules can decrease stress for mom and baby.

Chapter 7:

Establishing a Schedule for Baby

Humans love schedules, which decreases our anxiety and stress in our lives. So it is normal for mothers to want their babies to be on a schedule. We have to be realistic; all newborns are sleepy. As we have previously discussed, a baby must learn how to suck, swallow, and breathe as your milk supply increases. It is not practical to put a newborn on a schedule until your baby has learned to suck, swallow, and breath, your baby is less sleepy, and you have a full milk supply. I want to take you on baby's journey as he learns to breastfeed, from birth to the progression of establishing a feeding time, a playtime, and a nighttime schedule.

Your baby's journey of learning to breastfeed begins at birth. Let's start the baby's journey with his first latch after delivery; immediately after your baby is born, he is placed on your chest skin-to-skin. I know you may have read and expected your baby to latch onto your breast in the first hour after birth, but please do not worry if this does not occur. After delivery, while your baby is skin-to-skin, watch for any feeding cues, such as opening his eyes or hand-mouth activity. When you see a feeding cue, slowly lower the baby's mouth to the level of your nipple, allowing the baby to lick and nuzzle your nipple. This stimulation to the breast will cause your breast to leak colostrum. At every feeding cue, continue to alternate nipples so baby can lick, nuzzle, and possibly latch to receive drops of colostrum.

If your newborn does not show feeding cues, such as opening his eyes or hand-mouth activity every 2-3 hours, stimulate your baby and attempt to latch with assistance from the hospital's lactation consultant. If your baby is not latching every 2-3 hours, you need to hand express or pump and give your baby the colostrum by a curved tip or needle-less syringe. I want to take you through the steps of how to feed your baby by way of a syringe. You or your support person can hold your baby upright as if giving him a bottle. Intermittently squirt pumped colostrum into the corner of your baby's mouth and then remove the syringe from the baby's mouth to allow him to swallow. The baby will taste the milk and begin to suck and swallow as he receives food and calories. This bolus of colostrum will keep your baby's blood sugar elevated, preventing weight loss, dehydration, and jaundice. The increase in breast stimulation from pumping will increase milk production.

If your baby is not latching after being discharged from the hospital, the mother should call a lactation consultant for assistance. I recommend mothers attempt latching their baby with every feeding cue, such as opening his eyes, hand-mouth activity, or every 2-3 hours day and night. If your baby is not latching, pump your breasts for 15-20 minutes every 2-3 hours for adequate breast stimulation and milk production; continue to give the baby your pumped milk by a syringe. I would not give your baby more than 1-2 bottles a day until breastfeeding is more established at this learning stage. Early breast stimulation, by baby or pump, provides mom with long-term milk supply.

The question is, when do you put your baby on a schedule? The majority of mothers need to return to work approximately six weeks after delivery. Every new mother's goal is to decrease stress upon returning to work, and this begins with putting your baby on a schedule. Since you will be returning to work in 6 weeks, we have to give adequate time to increase milk production, introduce your baby to a bottle, and begin to practice putting your baby on a schedule. I would recommend starting a routine when your baby is around three weeks old. The best way to begin a schedule is to wake up your baby in the daytime, every 2 hours from the beginning of the last feeding, limiting the amount of daytime sleeping. To begin this process, I recommend slowly and gently waking up your baby using tummy time, placing the baby on the floor on a mat or blanket. During tummy time, massage and sing to your baby, intermittently turning him from back to front as he slowly wakes up. When you see your baby showing feeding cues, such as opening his eyes or hand-mouth activity, slowly take off his clothes down to the diaper, change his diaper, and breastfeed. After breastfeeding, pump for 15-20 minutes using your double electric breast pump. During the nighttime, allow your baby to wake up on his own; limited sleep in the daytime and exercise from tummy time will cause your baby to be more tired at night. Your baby will begin to sleep longer at night within a few weeks. Patients tell me that their baby is sleeping most of the night by six weeks old after following these instructions.

I feel that all adults need a bedtime routine; babies are no different. A bedtime routine should start in the evening at the most convenient time for your schedule; the average time is around 7–8 p.m. A bedtime routine begins with a warm bath, massage, bottle, pumping, and finally, bedtime. A warm bath and massage will increase relaxation to aid your baby to sleep. During the bath and massage, sing and enjoy this special time of bonding. After bath and massage, your support person will give the baby his bottle of pumped milk or formula; it is time for the baby to go to bed. As your support person gives your baby his bottle, you need to pump your breasts15-20 minutes with your double electric breast pump. After the bedtime routine, it is time for mommy to go to bed. A routine for napping and bedtime, with the same schedule day after day, will provide the baby with a sense of security. You are going to be surprised at how your baby will begin to love floor time (tummy time) and bath time.

Following these scheduled routines provides the baby with decreased sleeping time in the day and increased nighttime sleeping. Babies, children, and adults need adequate sleep for their mental and physical health. Establishing day and night routines has multiple benefits. Tummy time will teach your baby self-soothing and how to play independently. Introducing a bottle to your baby around three weeks of age will decrease stress to mom, baby, and babysitter. An increase in your pumping schedule will increase milk production, preparing for you to return to work. Another advantage of establishing scheduled routines is an increase in mommy time.

As we have previously discussed, stress and fear of the unknown can affect breastfeeding. The biggest fear of breastfeeding is the possibility of challenges or problems that could occur. In this next chapter, we will talk about difficulties in breastfeeding and the prevention and treatment of these problems.

Chapter 8:

Possible Breastfeeding Problems and Treatments

When I teach breastfeeding classes, I ask mothers what they have heard about breastfeeding. Mothers tell me breastfeeding is hard and painful. I feel sorry for mew moms; all they hear are the horror stories about breastfeeding. I can understand why mothers are scared to breastfeed. The best way to decrease fears of breastfeeding is to increase knowledge. This chapter will discuss the prevention and treatment of possible problems or challenges in breastfeeding mothers and babies. These challenges include sore nipples, bleb, engorgement, plugged ducts, mastitis, and yeast infections. Breastfeeding can be affected by mom or baby's anatomy issues, such as flat and inverted nipples of the mother and problems with the baby's mouth or tongue. Milk supply is critical in breastfeeding. We are going to talk about reasons for low milk supply and an oversupply of breast milk. I will discuss how the color, taste, and smell of foods and drinks can affect your breast milk. I hope that discussing possible breastfeeding challenges and problems will decrease your fear. When your fear is reduced, you and your baby will be more relaxed, resulting in an enjoyable feeding. I want to begin our discussion with the most common problem or challenge in breastfeeding, sore nipples.

SORE NIPPLES

Before we discuss sore nipples, I want to review some myths mothers may hear concerning sore nipples. The first myth is that mothers need to toughen their nipples in pregnancy before breastfeeding; this is not true. Mothers do not need to rub or toughen their nipples in pregnancy, preparing to breastfeed. When you and your baby are comfortable, and the baby is latched correctly, you will not have pain. Another myth is that pain on the nipples is normal when you and your baby are learning to breastfeed; this is not true. Pain when you are breastfeeding means you should stop and get assistance from a lactation consultant. If you are having pain with latching baby onto your breast, you must not wait to ask for help. Postponing assistance from a lactation consultant will increase damage to your nipples, increasing pain; affect breastfeeding. Another myth that moms commonly hear is that breastfeeding always hurts at the start of the feeding; this is not true. Pain with latching baby onto your breast at the beginning of the feeding is a signal you need to break the seal of baby's suck, go slowly, take your time, and re-latch baby. If you attempt to re-latch your baby and pain persists, you need to call a lactation consultant for assistance. Let's discuss some reasons mothers may develop sore nipples.

I feel the main reason mothers have sore nipples is from a poor latch, most commonly caused by poor positioning. In the newborn stage, inadequate support to the baby's head and neck can cause nipples to be sore. If you are having pain with latching your baby onto your breasts in the hospital, it is imperative to ask for assistance from a lactation consultant. If pain with latching continues after discharge from the hospital, you need to call a lactation consultant for evaluation and assistance.

Let's talk about how moisture can affect your nipples. When you lick your lips, they become chapped from the moisture. When moisture is left on your nipples, like your lips, they may become chapped and possibly crack or open. To prevent nipple chapping, keep your nipples dry. Get into the habit of patting your nipples dry after each feeding or pumping.

Another common reason for sore nipples is repeatedly pulling the baby off your breast when your baby is sleeping at the breast or having pain while breastfeeding. The baby has a strong seal from the suction he has on your breast. Pulling baby off of your breasts, over and over, causes rubbing or abrasions on the nipples. To prevent sore nipples, always place your finger into the corner of your baby's mouth, break the seal of his suck, and remove him from your breast.

Mothers often ask me if they can wash their breasts. Soap can cause your nipples to become dry and eventually cause your nipples to crack and become sore. Yes, you can take a shower but rinse your nipples with soapy water; do not directly wash them with soap. As discussed earlier, soap can also dry up the anti-bacterial oil on the Montgomery glands located on your areola.

When you are preparing to return to work, you need to evaluate if the flange, the cone-shaped part of the breast pump that fits your areola, is the right size. A flange that is too small or too large can cause pressure and irritation on your nipples and areola; if you are having pain with pumping, call your breast pump manufacturer and discuss how your flange fits. A representative will recommend the correct size for the flange.

Some moms may have nipple pain from a condition called Raynaud's phenomenon. The mother's main complaint with Raynauds is pain on the nipples when her nipples are exposed to room air after she breastfeeds, which is cooler than the baby's mouth. This drop in temperature causes the nipples to spasm and can sometimes cause the nipples to appear white or blue after breastfeeding. Raynaud's phenomenon can be triggered by damage to the nipples from a poor latch or a yeast infection on the nipples. If trauma or yeast is the reason for Raynaud's, the pain should resolve after your nipples are treated and healed.[11] To decrease pain caused by spasms of your nipples, keep your nipples warm. In my experience, during

---

11 Gaskin Ina May : Ina May's Guide to Breastfeeding Bantam Books New York, New York 2009 Page 172-173

breastfeeding, I have mothers keep the opposite nipple covered as the baby feeds. Mothers I have assisted have had good results decreasing nipple pain by using a warm cloth on each nipple or a hairdryer on low after feeding; both treatments can be used for 2-3 minutes. Another treatment mothers can use to decrease spasms caused by a drop in the nipples' temperature is to apply a warm microwavable relief pack inside her bra after feeding. There are multiple treatments to dilate blood vessels on the nipple preventing pain. Besides heat, a medication that dilates blood vessels on the nipples called nifedipine can be useful to decrease nipple spasms and pain; a prescription is needed from your ob-gyn. As recommended per Dr. Jack Newman, Vitamin B6 can be effective for pain on the nipples caused by Raynaud's spasms.[12]

Prevention is the key to treating sore nipples. After delivery, it is vital to ask for assistance from a lactation consultant in the hospital if you are having pain from a poor latch. Early intervention of a poor latch can prevent sore, cracked, bleeding nipples. If you have sore nipples, I recommend starting each feeding on the nipple that is less painful, as the baby is hungry and sucks harder on the first breast. It can be very soothing to apply a warm, moist compress with a washcloth to your breast 3-4 times a day for 2-3 minutes; a perfect time is when you go to the bathroom. After the application of a warm, moist compress, air-dry your nipples to promote healing. It is crucial after you breastfeed or pump to pat -dry or air-dry your nipples and apply expressed breast milk, coconut oil (if not allergic), or lanolin cream (if not allergic to wool) to moisturize your nipples and prevent dryness. If your nipples are cracked, or the skin opens, it is essential to use an over-the-counter antibiotic ointment. The antibiotic ointment will prevent bacteria from entering through the cracks and traveling to the milk ducts, possibly causing a bacterial infection (mastitis) or a yeast infection. You can gently remove the ointment before breastfeeding with a warm washcloth. A great ointment for your nipples is All-Purpose

12 Newman Jack MD and Pitman Teresa the Ultimate Breastfeeding Book Of Answers
    Three Rivers Press New York, New York 2006 Page 104-106

Nipple Ointment (APNO) by Dr. Jack Newman; it contains an antibiotic, an antifungal, and an anti-inflammatory. According to Dr. Newman, you do not need to wipe APNO off of your breasts before breastfeeding. Please be aware that you will need a prescription from your ob-gyn for APNO ointment. APNO is made of multiple ingredients and needs to be filled at a compounding pharmacy; the pharmacist mixes one or more medications for the prescribed medication (Like mixing ingredients for a cake). Do not worry about finding a compounding pharmacy; they are in every city for physicians to order prescriptions to meet all patients' needs.

FLAT AND INVERTED NIPPLES

As I have previously mentioned, all breasts, nipples, and areolas are different; the shape and appearance of your nipples may affect breastfeeding; this is one reason nipples should be examined at the prenatal visits. Mothers need to be prepared for the possibility of needing assistance from a lactation consultant, after delivery, for flat or inverted nipples. Your nipple is in the center of your areola and is usually slightly raised and erect. Nipples that are not erect and lay flat, even with the areola, are called *flat nipples*. Nipples that appear to be pulling inward instead of sticking out are called *inverted nipples*. Inverted nipples are caused by adhesions at the base of the nipples that bind the skin to the underlying tissue, preventing nipples from sticking outward.

With flat or inverted nipples, your baby may or may not have difficulty latching due to your nipples not being erect. I want to discuss some treatment measures that may help your baby latch onto your breast with flat or inverted nipples. I recommend wearing a breast shell starting at 38 weeks of pregnancy, during the daytime. A breast shell is a plastic disk consisting of two pieces, a base and a dome. The dome has a hole in the center that applies pressure to the base or bottom of your nipple, causing the nipple to protrude through the hole and slowly stretch adhesions. After delivery, use the breast shell 1-2 hours before breastfeeding, as prolonged use can cause engorgement.

With flat and inverted nipples, I recommend pumping your breasts for 5 minutes before you breastfeed to stretch adhesions. After pumping, perform exercises to pull out your nipple. An exercise called reverse pressure softening can be useful in pulling your nipple out. To perform this exercise, use one of your hands and circle the base of your nipple with your fingertips and the tip of your thumb. With your fingertips and the end of your thumb, apply pressure inward, toward your chest wall, for 1-3 minutes to stretch adhesions.[13] Before latching your baby onto your breast, roll your nipple between your fingers to keep the nipple sticking out for an easier latch. After breastfeeding, pump your breasts for 10-15 minutes to stretch adhesions and slowly pull your nipple outward. In time you will be able to decrease exercises and pumping as the adhesions stretch and your nipples begin to stick out. Remember, every mother is different. These treatment measures may not be effective for all mothers, or the treatment measures may take different amounts of time to erect the nipples.

Latching baby onto your breast can be a challenge with flat or inverted nipples. A breast hold called the 'breast sandwich technique' can be very useful in assisting your baby to latch.

The step-by-step process of performing the breast sandwich technique

- Position one hand on your breast, resembling a 'C 'shape
- Place your thumb above your breast and your fingers below your breast at the edge of the areola
- Compress your fingers and thumb gently together, pushing back towards your chest wall; this narrows the areola and provides more breast tissue, making it easier for your baby to latch.

---

13 Mohrbacherb Nancy , Breastfeeding Answers Made Simple Hale Publishing Amarillo, Texas 2010 Page 796

[14]If your baby cannot latch using a 'breast sandwich technique, a nipple shield can be effective for flat or inverted nipples. Using a nipple shield will gradually pull on flat nipples, causing them to stick out. It also works well for inverted nipples, gradually breaking adhesions, pulling the nipples out. The mother should attempt to latch the baby without a nipple shield, using the' breast sandwich' hold, every few days.

BLEB

If you notice a small, painful, white, or yellow pimple on your nipple, this is a bleb. It occurs when the skin has grown over the milk duct opening or pore. When you see a bleb on your nipple, you need to determine the cause of the bleb. The most common reason for a bleb is from pinching or rubbing the nipples from a poor latch, incorrect flange size of your breast pump, or incorrect placement or size of a nipple shield.

As with sore nipples, prevention is the key. If you have pain or pinching from a poor latch, you need to call a lactation consultant. If you feel pain or rubbing when you pump, contact your breast pump manufacturer to be evaluated for a different size flange. A pinching feeling when using a nipple shield needs to be assessed by a lactation consultant to verify you are applying the nipple shield correctly and using the correct size.

A bleb feels hard to the touch and will need to be softened to allow the area to open and heal. The best way to soften a bleb is to apply heat. Before breastfeeding, you can use a variety of heat treatments to soften the bleb, such as using a heating pad on low for 20-30 minutes to the area of the bleb, rubbing the bleb with a washcloth in a warm shower, applying a warm, moist compress with a washcloth, or breast therapy warm relief packs. After the heat treatment, pump your breasts for 5 minutes to attempt to open the bleb. Breastfeed on the affected breast first, since the baby is hungry and will pull harder to open the bleb. After breastfeeding,

---

14 www.askdrsears.com

use a cotton ball with extra virgin olive oil to soften the bleb. Extra virgin olive oil has healing and anti-inflammatory properties.[15]

After the bleb has opened, apply a small amount of over-the-counter antibiotic ointment to the area; remove ointment before breastfeeding with a warm washcloth. Expose the nipple to air as much as possible to promote healing. Again, a great ointment to use after the bleb opens is APNO; it contains an antibiotic and an anti-inflammatory. As we discussed in treating sore nipples, a prescription for APNO is needed from your ob-gyn.

ENGORGEMENT

Engorgement is when your breasts become full of milk, and your milk ducts are distended from excessive milk production. Engorgement is normal and occurs around 3-4 days after birth. Your breasts will be swollen, slightly pink to light red, and warm to the touch. You may see and feel swelling and lumps under your armpits, where your milk line begins.

The best treatment for engorgement is breastfeeding, but sometimes your breasts are very firm, and the baby has difficulty latching. Heat therapy is the best treatment to soften the breasts and make it earlier for your baby to latch. Before breastfeeding, you can use various heat treatments to soften the breasts, such as using a heating pad on low for 20-30 minutes, taking a warm shower with massage, applying warm, moist compresses with a washcloth, or breast therapy warm relief packs. Heat treatment using your fingers to massage under your armpits may help soften and loosen the milk inside the distended milk ducts along the milk line. After heat treatment, I recommend pumping with breast massage for 5 minutes to soften your areola and help your baby latch.

---

15 Jayne Leonard Medical News Today Article Name: How Do You Treat a Milk Blister? May 3 2018

The step-by-step process of performing breast massage:

- Position one hand on your breast, resembling a 'C 'shape

- Place your thumb above your breast and your fingers below your breast, not touching the areola

- Slide your thumb and fingers together towards your nipple, stopping at the edge of the areola

- Repeat as needed

Another breast massage technique is to use your fingers to make circular motions around your entire breast, similar to performing a self-breast exam. As discussed in the treatment of flat or inverted nipples, reverse pressure softening can make it easier for the baby to latch.

During engorgement, your baby's stomach will become full faster due to the excessive milk inside of your milk ducts. After breastfeeding, feel your breasts for any hard areas; if you feel lumps or hard areas, this is retained milk in your milk ducts that your baby could not remove during the feeding. To remove the retained milk in your milk ducts, pump your breasts for 10 minutes after breastfeeding. The length of time you will need to pump will depend on your comfort and how full your breasts feel. After pumping, you can use various cold or ice treatments for swelling and discomfort, such as chilled, washed cabbage leaves inside your bra, bags of frozen vegetables such as peas or corn, or breast therapy cold packs inside your bra. Cold therapy treatments can be used for 10 minutes after each feeding or what time frame is comfortable for you; limit the use of cabbage leaves to 10 minutes 2 times a day to prevent a decrease in milk supply. You can take ibuprofen (Advil) for pain and inflammation if you are not allergic. During engorgement, avoid nipple stimulation with intercourse and wear a bra to bed to prevent an increase in milk supply.

PLUGGED DUCTS

If you feel a hard area on your breast after breastfeeding, this is called a plugged milk duct. This hardened area results from retained milk inside your milk duct that your baby could not remove during the feeding. It is vital to recognize and treat plugged ducts. Make it a habit to feel your breasts after each feeding for hard areas. If you feel a pea-, dime-, or nickel-sized area, do not ignore it. A plugged duct will feel tender, warm, and appear slightly red. You may develop a low-grade fever and have mild chills.

What are the causes of plugged ducts? Ask yourself, is your baby latching well, or is he falling asleep at the breast? Do you have an over-production of milk, making it difficult for your baby to empty your milk ducts when he feeds? If your baby is sleepy, he needs an increase in stimulation to stay awake and breastfeed. If your baby has a poor latch or you have an overproduction of breast milk, you need to call a lactation consultant for evaluation and treatment.

To avoid plugged ducts, I do not recommend feeding your baby at a scheduled time or skipping a feeding. Breastfeeding your baby at a scheduled time can cause milk to remain inside your milk ducts for an extended time; the retained milk will become thick and hard and develop into plugged ducts. Try not to skip a feeding; if you realize you need to miss a feeding, pump your breasts in the place of that feeding to avoid retained milk in the milk ducts, preventing plugged ducts. It is essential to feed your baby or pump your breasts every 2-3 hours or per your baby's feeding cues. To prevent constriction and blocking of your milk ducts, avoid bras that are too small or with wire support, and avoid prolonged pressure of a heavy purse or diaper bag on your breasts.

To compress the hard areas on your breast and soften the milk inside your milk ducts, you can rotate breastfeeding positions such as cross-cradle or football. As previously discussed in chapter five, breast compression can increase your breast's stimulation and increase milk production; an added advantage is it effectively softens your plugged ducts. Breast massage can soften your areola and help your baby latch when your breasts are engorged, can also soften, and remove the hardened milk inside the milk duct.

The treatment of plugged ducts consists of measures to loosen and soften the hardened milk inside your milk duct. Heat treatments can be beneficial in softening the hardened milk inside of the milk duct. Before breastfeeding, use various heat treatments, such as a warm shower, a heating pad on low applied to the affected area for 20-30 minutes, use a warm, moist compress with a washcloth to the affected area, or breast therapy warm relief packs. Breast massage or breast compression can be used in the shower and before and during breastfeeding; to soften and loosen the hardened milk. Breastfeed on the affected breast first, since the baby is hungry and will pull harder to loosen the milk. After breastfeeding, pump for 5-10 minutes, with breast massage or breast compression, to continue to loosen and remove the milk. As recommended per Dr. Jack Newman, Lecithin, a food additive, reduces breast milk stickiness by preventing fats from clumping together, decreasing plugged ducts.[16]

MASTITIS

Mastitis results from milk remaining inside the milk duct that has become bigger, harder, and has grown bacteria, causing an infection. The mastitis symptoms are a hard area that is red, very tender, and very warm to the touch. You will have flu-like symptoms, including fever, chills, and tiredness. Prevention is the key to mastitis; feel your breasts after each feeding for any hard area, do not ignore plugged ducts. To prevent mastitis, like preventing plugged ducts, avoid scheduled or timed feedings, and avoid skipping a feeding.

The treatment of mastitis has the same goal as plugged ducts, to soften the hardened milk inside your milk duct. Heat with massage is

16 Newman Jack MD and Pitman Theresa The Ultimate Breastfeeding Book of Answers Three Rivers Press New York, New York 2000 Page 126

effective in softening the hardened milk. Before breastfeeding, use various heat treatments, such as a warm shower with gentle massage, use a heating pad on low applied to the affected area for 20-30 minutes. Apply warm, moist compresses with a washcloth to the affected area or breast therapy warm relief packs. Breastfeed on the affected breast first since the baby is hungry and will pull harder to loosen the hardened milk. After breastfeeding, pump for 5-10 minutes, with gentle massage, to soften and remove the milk. After pumping, you can use various cold or ice treatments for swelling and discomfort, such as chilled, washed cabbage leaves inside your bra, bags of frozen vegetables such as peas or corn, or breast therapy cold packs inside your bra. Cold therapy treatments can be used for 10 minutes after each feeding or what time frame is comfortable for you.

You can take ibuprofen for fever, chills, and pain, if not allergic. You need to call your ob-gyn with any signs of mastitis. Your ob-gyn will treat you with an antibiotic since mastitis is an infection. He will order an antibiotic that is approved and safe to take while breastfeeding. Until mastitis has resolved, avoid nipple stimulation with intercourse and wear a bra to bed to prevent an increase in milk supply

YEAST

You might not realize you can get a yeast infection on your nipples. Yeast is an overgrowth of fungus that loves to grow in moist, dark places. You would not believe where yeast can grow, on your nipples, feet, mouth, vagina, baby's buttocks, and even your pet's ears. How do you know if you have a yeast infection? One of the first signs of a yeast infection is burning red, itchy, tender, and flakey nipples when you are breastfeeding. If your baby is latching well, but you have pain on your nipples when you are breastfeeding, yeast may be causing the pain. Sharp shooting pains, like glass, through your breast during and after feeding can indicate that yeast has spread into your milk ducts. You can continue to breastfeed with a yeast infection, but you need to call and discuss these symptoms with a lactation consultant and your ob-gyn for evaluation and treatment.

Can your baby get a yeast infection? Yes, if you have a yeast infection, your baby must be treated, even if he does not have any symptoms. If the baby is not treated, the yeast infection will continue to pass back and forth from mom to baby. Signs of a yeast infection in a baby are increased gas, an increase in fussiness, and baby pulling on and off the breast. Yeast may cause your baby to develop thrush or white patches inside his mouth, gums, and cheeks. If the mother has yeast symptoms on her breasts, the baby should be treated, even if the pediatrician cannot see white patches in the baby's mouth. If your baby has a red, raised rash on his buttocks, he may have a yeast diaper rash and needs to be treated with an antifungal cream. To prevent yeast growth on your baby's bottom, make it a habit to always pat the area dry after each diaper change.

Can you give your baby pumped milk when you have a yeast infection? Yes, you can give your baby freshly pumped breast milk, as long as you and baby are being treated for yeast. Yeast is not killed in the breast milk by refrigeration or freezing.

Preventing yeast growth on your nipples and areola is very important, so always air-dry or pat dry your nipples after each feeding and pumping. I encourage moms to keep clean breast pads available and to change them when they are damp. Do not wear your gym clothes or a wet bathing suit for a prolonged period; to prevent the growth of a vaginal yeast infection. Believe it or not, tight jeans and pantyhose can increase moisture, increasing yeast growth in the vaginal area. Please be sure you wash your hands well before handling the baby, breastfeeding, or pumping to prevent yeast from spreading to your baby. A family member with athletes' feet should wear socks and wash their hands before handling the baby. If yeast infections are recurrent, consider having your cat's or dog's ears checked by their veterinarian. Be aware some medications can cause yeast to grow, including antibiotics, birth control pills, prednisone, and other steroids.

If you suspect that you or your baby has a yeast infection, call your ob-gyn and pediatrician for evaluation and treatment. Your pediatrician will prescribe an oral antifungal suspension that should be painted on the baby's tongue, the roof of his mouth, and the sides or cheeks of his mouth. Your doctor will prescribe an antifungal cream (such as nystatin, clotrimazole, miconazole) for your nipples.[17] If your healthcare provider advises you to wash the creams off your nipples before breastfeeding, do so gently with warm water. APNO, which is an antifungal, can also be prescribed to treat yeast on your nipples. As Dr. Jack Newman recommends, you do not need to wipe APNO off your nipples before breastfeeding. Coconut oil is also an excellent antifungal and is safe for breastfeeding if you are not allergic. Yeast organisms hate sunlight. Expose your nipples to sunlight 1-2 times a day, after applying an antifungal solution of diluted vinegar with a cotton ball, using 1 cup of water to 2 tablespoons of white vinegar. Yeast can live on any item that comes in contact with the baby's mouth or your nipples. Once a day, it is recommended to soak pump parts, nipples, bottles, and pacifiers in a sink of hot water with a diluted vinegar solution (1-2 cups of white vinegar), wash pump parts after soaking, rinse parts well, and completely dry. Wear 100 % cotton bras and wash them daily in vinegar and hot water.

A change in diet may help prevent yeast. Eat yogurt with live active cultures, which encourages good bacteria to live in your gut, reducing yeast growth. Consider decreasing sugar in your diet, which increases the growth of yeast. Discuss the use of probiotics with your ob-gyn. Probiotics, acidophilus, are live microbial organisms that are naturally present in the digestive tract and vagina. They are referred to as friendly bacteria and help suppress the growth of organisms, including yeast.

Yeast infections can be very persistent, so take the full course of medication suggested by your doctor and baby's pediatrician. Continue using the home remedies for 2-3 weeks so that the infection will not reoccur.

---

17 Hale, Thomas PhD and Pamela Berens MD Clinical Therapy in Breastfeeding Patients Hale Publishing Amarillo, Texas 2002 Page 95

TONGUE- THRUSTING

Some newborns play with their tongue and make a clicking sound; these babies may be tongue- thrusting; a condition that begins when your baby is still in your uterus, finds his tongue, lifts his tongue to the roof of his mouth, and sucks on it like a pacifier. When your baby lifts his tongue to the roof of his mouth, it has a significant effect on breastfeeding. After your baby is born and you attempt to latch the baby onto your breast, your breast tissue will block him from lifting his tongue. In response, your baby will become frustrated, he will refuse to latch, and he will shake his head from side to side and scream; keep in mind that your baby has been sucking on his tongue in utero, which provided him with comfort and security. After your baby is born, he will want to continue to suck on his tongue for comfort and security as he is adjusting to his new world. A baby is very smart and will slide down to the tip of your nipple to lift his tongue to the roof of his mouth, causing pinching of your nipples and severe nipple pain. When your baby is sucking on the tip of your nipple, he appears to be latched because he is moving his mouth; this is one reason mothers are told in the hospital that their baby is latched well. The mother is confused if her baby is latched well, why is the latch on her breast so painful. Many mothers suffer for weeks because tongue-thrusting has not been diagnosed; thus, the mother has received inadequate breast stimulation and now has a decreased milk supply. When babies tongue thrust, the mothers feel chopping or biting on her nipples during breastfeeding, resulting in red, purple, or lipstick-shaped nipples. Weight loss is common with these babies because the mother and lactation consultants believe the baby is latching. It is very important to verify your baby is swallowing and receiving milk. Tongue-thrusting babies struggle with bottle-feeding; when mom attempts to give her baby a bottle, he will lift his tongue, making it difficult for the baby to suck and swallow; this is why moms see milk dripping from the baby's mouth when she bottle- feeds her baby.

How do you prevent tongue-thrusting babies from lifting their tongue? The first treatment I use to assist tongue-thrusting babies to suck with their tongue down is using a nipple shield. A baby will tolerate the shield because he can still feel some of his tongue. Using a nipple shield, the baby becomes more comfortable at the breast; the mother receives increased breast stimulation, increasing milk supply. Another exercise is to hold a pacifier in the baby's mouth for 5 minutes before each feeding and throughout the day when your baby is awake. Training your baby to suck with his tongue down can take 1-3 weeks or longer.

If your baby is tongue-thrusting and you determine you have a decreased milk supply, pumping after breastfeeding and supplementation with formula may be needed. The need to pump or supplement will depend on your milk supply and your baby's feeding cues.

LOW MILK SUPPLY

Milk supply is critical in breastfeeding. There are times when a mother has a low milk supply for a variety of reasons. Before I discuss the causes of low milk supply, I want to discuss how to recognize a low milk supply and review a suggested breastfeeding and pumping schedule to increase your milk supply.

What are the signs of a decreased milk supply? One of the first signs of a decreased milk supply is the absence of baby swallowing. Watch your baby; he will respond to a decreased milk supply by pulling away from the breast. With a decreased milk supply baby will turn his head during the feeding, appear uncomfortable during the feeding, be fussy between and after feeding, and sleep poorly due to hunger. If your baby is not receiving adequate food, he will lose weight, he will have decreased wet diapers and bowel movements, and he may become dehydrated and develop jaundice.

If you determine you have a decreased milk supply, what can you do? Let's discuss a schedule to increase milk supply, including breastfeeding, supplementation with formula, and a pumping schedule for day and night time feedings.

Daytime feeding: The following schedule should be used:

- Breastfeed your baby per feeding cues, such as fussiness, opening his eyes, hand-mouth activity, or every 2-3 hours. As your baby is nursing your support person, using a curved tip or need-less syringe will intermittently squirt pumped milk or formula into the corner of your baby's mouth. Your baby will taste the milk and want to suck harder, increasing breast stimulation and milk production. I recommend breastfeeding 5-7 minutes on each breast due to low milk supply. The frequency of rotating your breast will increase as your milk supply increases. The use of a syringe will decrease as your milk supply increases.

- Supplement your baby with 1-2 ounces of formula and observe your baby for signs his stomach is full; he will be appearing relaxed and not showing any hunger cues. If your baby is showing feeding or hunger cues, increase the amount of formula.

- Pump your breasts after breastfeeding for 15-20 minutes to increase breast stimulation and your milk supply.

Nighttime feeding: The following schedule should be used:

- Breastfeed your baby per feeding cues, such as fussiness, opening his eyes, hand-mouth activity, or every 3 hours. As your baby is nursing your support person, using a curved tip or need-less syringe will intermittently squirt pumped milk or formula into the corner of the baby's mouth. I recommend breastfeeding 5-7 minutes on each breast due to low milk supply.

- Supplement your baby with 1-2 ounces of formula and observe your baby for signs his stomach is full; he will be appearing relaxed and not showing any hunger cues. If your baby is showing feeding or hunger cues, increase the amount of formula.

- Pump your breasts after breastfeeding for 10-15 minutes instead of 15-20 minutes to enable you to get more rest during the night for your physical and mental health

You can also add power pumping to your schedule for a faster increase in your milk supply. Power pumping consists of pumping for 30 minutes with massage (massage your breasts 1-2 minutes, pump 10 minutes, massage your breasts 1-2 minutes, pump 10 minutes, massage your breasts 1-2 minutes, pump 10 minutes). I recommend power pumping twice a day, in the morning after the first feeding of the day and the evening before bed. There are various ways to power pump your breasts; I have found this particular schedule helpful for mothers. While you are pumping, you can listen to music you love to sing or watch your favorite funny movie to increase relaxation and promote your milk let-down.

These methods of increasing your milk production are a win-win situation. Using a syringe with pumped milk or formula while your baby is breastfeeding increases the baby's security and comfort on your breasts. Supplementation with formula provides the baby with nutrition, and pumping increases your breast milk production. A syringe is used for approximately 5-7 days until breast milk has increased and your baby is breastfeeding effectively. Within 7-10 days, the baby is fully breastfeeding with little to no supplementation with formula, and the need for power pumping has decreased.

Studies show breast massage and breast compression can increase breast milk output; it is advantageous to massage your breast before and during breastfeeding and pumping. I want you to understand the purpose of breast massage and breast compression is to soften the hardened milk inside your milk ducts, increase the milk flow through the milk ducts, emptying your milk ducts; increasing milk output. These massage techniques do not have to be performed perfectly; as long as you apply pressure to your milk ducts, that is comfortable for you.[18]

Milk production is critical in breastfeeding. Some mothers cannot produce an adequate milk supply for a variety of reasons. I want to discuss the reasons that some mothers may have a low milk supply.

A poor latch onto your breast is one of the main reasons for a decrease in milk supply. An ineffective latch results in inadequate stimulation to your breasts, resulting in low milk supply. If your baby has a poor latch, it is essential to consult with a lactation consultant for evaluation and treatment.

A variety of medical issues with mom can affect prolactin, the milk-making hormone, and oxytocin, the hormone that causes the milk to let-down into your milk ducts. A medical condition that can affect milk production is diabetes, which causes the mother to have insulin resistance. The mammary gland, which makes milk, is dependent upon insulin. I recommend mothers with diabetes begin pumping their breasts on the day of delivery 10-15 minutes after each feeding with every feeding cue of their baby, such as opening his eyes, hand-mouth activity, or every 2-3 hours. It is important that these mothers are followed by a lactation consultant to monitor the baby's weight, monitor the baby's output of wet and bowel movements, and monitor the mother's milk supply. Problems with a mother's thyroid gland can also affect milk production. The thyroid gland, found in the front of your neck, secretes hormones that regulate prolactin and oxytocin. Mothers diagnosed with hypothyroidism (Hashimoto's Disease) may notice hair loss, dry skin, and decreased milk supply. Mothers diagnosed with hyperthyroid (Grave's Disease) may have an increased heart rate, fine, brittle hair, problems with the let-down of their milk, and an oversupply of breast milk. I recommend mothers with hypothyroid begin pumping their breasts on the day of delivery 10-15 minutes after each feeding with every

---

18 Mohrbacher Nancy , 2010 Breastfeeding Answers Made Simple. A Guide Helping
    Mothers. Amarillo, TX, Hale Publishing Page 417, 468

feeding cue of their baby, such as opening his eyes, hand-mouth activity, or every 2-3 hours. Mothers with hyperthyroid may have an overproduction of breast milk with a fast let-down; please refer to the treatments of the overproduction of breast milk. Discuss with your ob-gyn if you have a history of diabetes or symptoms of hypothyroid or hyperthyroid.

During your pregnancy, you need to discuss with your ob-gyn if you have a polycystic ovarian disorder (PCOS), enlarged ovaries with cysts, causing a hormone imbalance. Mothers with PCOS have elevated androgens, male hormones, which interfere with the production and function of estrogen, prolactin, and oxytocin. Estrogen is responsible for developing breast tissue or glandular tissue, prolactin is responsible for milk production, and oxytocin is responsible for milk let-down. Every woman is different, and the degree of symptoms can vary from mom to mom. Do not assume that because you have PCOS, you will not be able to breastfeed. It is essential that these mothers are followed by a lactation consultant to monitor the baby's weight, monitor the baby's output of wet and bowel movements, and monitor the mother's milk supply

Stress can affect your milk supply. Sometimes we do not realize how stressed we are at different times in our life. One of the most stressful times for a woman is during and after delivering her baby; it is happy, joyful, but stressful. Stress releases a hormone called cortisol, which decreases milk let-down and ultimately decreases milk production. A simple way to decrease stress, to prevent a decrease in milk production is relaxation and visualization. Relaxing with breathing, music, or meditation can reduce your stress and anxiety. Believe it or not, when you visualize your milk flowing or a happy memory, you feel relaxed, increasing the let-down of your milk into your milk ducts. Your baby will respond to your increase in milk flow by sucking harder, emptying your milk ducts, increasing milk supply.

Smoking cigarettes or using nicotine affects oxytocin and prolactin levels. Prolactin is responsible for milk production, and oxytocin is responsible for milk let-down. As a result of smoking cigarettes, milk production, and the let-down of your milk can be affected, resulting in early weaning.

Some medications can affect your milk production. A few examples of medications that can decrease your milk supply are birth control pills containing estrogen, throat lozenges containing menthol, and decongestants.

Foods can affect milk production. Let's discuss various foods, beverages, and herbs that you should avoid that may cause a decrease in your milk supply such as, sage, jasmine tea, parsley, peppermint, and drinking alcoholic beverages. Alcoholic beverages can decrease the let-down of your milk and change the taste of your milk. Some babies do not like the taste of alcohol and will not breastfeed well, reducing your breasts' stimulation, decreasing your milk supply.[19]

Many cultures claim that certain foods, drinks, spices, and herbs increase milk supply; these are called galactagogues. They act on the pituitary gland, the part of the brain that increases prolactin production, which increases breast milk production. Galactagogues can help increase milk supply, but they do not work independently; they work in combination with breastfeeding and pumping to provide stimulation to your breasts. If you decide to take galactagogues, discuss the usage with your ob-gyn concerning any interaction with a medication or medical condition. These are a few galactagogues that may help to increase your milk supply.

- Foods that can act as galactagogues include dates, oatmeal, carrots, beets, yams, apricots, green papaya, nuts, grains, dark green leafy vegetables, seeds, legumes, flaxseeds, and lactation cookies. When taking papaya, be cautious if allergic to latex.

- Spices such as garlic, ginger, dill, cilantro, caraway, turmeric, anise, fennel, brewer's yeast can act as galactagogues.

19 Younger Meek Joan , MD RD FAAP IBCLC Mew Mothers Guide to Breastfeeding Bantam Trade Paperbacks New York, New York 2011 page 140

- Drinks including sports drinks, barley water (made with whole grains and pearl barley), non-alcoholic beer, teas such as Yogi, Milkmaid, and Organic Mothers Milk Tea can also be useful to aid in increasing milk supply.

- Certain herbs can act as galactagogues to increase your milk supply. More Milk Plus, produced by a company called Motherlove, contains the herbs fenugreek, blessed thistle, nettle, fennel, goats rue (increases breast tissue), and alfalfa leaf (caution if allergic to peanuts or have a clotting issue).[20] A galactagogue called Go-Lacta, which contains an herb called Moringa, may also help improve your milk supply. These herbs are not taken together; take one or the other.

OVER- PRODUCTION OF BREASTMILK

Milk production is necessary for breastfeeding, but the oversupply of breast milk can affect your baby nursing. Overproduction of milk supply can begin in the first 2-3 weeks postpartum but can occur at any time. A sign of an oversupply of breast milk can be when you observe your baby gagging, choking, and pulling away from your breasts as he is breastfeeding, caused by a fast let-down of your milk into his mouth. As a result, your baby may have an increase in fussiness, gas, and colic symptoms, which causes an increase of air entering into his stomach. The fast let-down of your milk may cause your baby to have shorter feedings, resulting in your baby's bowel movements changing to a green color, which indicates the baby receiving too much foremilk. The gaging, choking feeling from the fast let-down of your milk may cause your baby to refuse or reject your breast.

The goal of treating an oversupply of breast milk is to decrease breast milk production to reduce your discomfort and decrease the baby's difficulty swallowing related to your milk's fast flow. I recommend breastfeeding

---

20 Jacobson Hilary, Mother Food, food and herbs that promote milk production and a mother's health Rosalind Press Lexington Kentucky 2013 Chapter 20 page 256-300

in an upright, semi-sitting, or football position to reduce gagging or choking. Before breastfeeding, to prevent milk from squirting down your baby's throat, briefly hand massage or pump until you feel or see the let-down of your milk. To decrease stimulation to your breast, which will decrease milk supply, breastfeed on only one breast per feeding. During breastfeeding, if the baby attempts to go to sleep, break the seal of his suck, and stimulate him. Continue feeding on the SAME breast until the baby is content and not showing any feeding or hunger cues. On the opposite breast, if you are uncomfortable, briefly pump for 3-5 minutes. After breastfeeding, you can use a variety of ice treatments for discomfort, including bags of frozen vegetables such as peas or corn or breast therapy cold packs inside your bra. Ice therapy can be used, if needed, for 5-10 minutes or what time frame is comfortable for you. Usually, within 5-7 days, milk production has decreased; you can resume rotating breasts doing the feeding when your baby shows signs of going to sleep. Avoid nipple stimulation with intercourse and wear a bra to bed to prevent an increase in milk supply. Consult with your ob-gyn for the possibility of hyperthyroid if you continue to have an oversupply of your breast milk.

BREASTMILK: SOAPY OR METALLIC TASTE AND SMELL

If you notice your breast milk has a soapy or metallic taste and smell, it is not harmful to your baby. This change in the taste and smell of your breast milk can occur if you have an overproduction of lipase, an enzyme present in breast milk. Lipase breaks down the fats in the breast milk for easier absorption by your baby.

The bad taste and smell of breast milk increase with freezing. To prevent this from occurring, treat the breast milk by scalding your milk immediately after pumping. Scalding breast milk slows down or stops the breaking down of fats in the milk. To scald your milk, place milk in a pot, heat it until you see bubbles at the edge of the pot, cool milk, and then freeze milk. Do not bring the milk to a full boil.[21] Another option to decrease your milk's metallic or soapy taste and smell is to modify your diet. It is recommended to increase antioxidants, such as beta carotene and vitamin E, and avoid polyunsaturated fats, such as fish oil, flax seeds, anchovies, and vegetable oil.

LEAKING OF YOUR BREASTMILK

It can be very embarrassing when breast milk leaks through your clothes. Leaking breasts are common 3-4 days after birth when your milk ducts are full of milk. The leaking of your breasts may occur when you hear your baby cry or another baby cry, think about your baby, or smell your baby. If you feel your breasts leaking and are unable to nurse or pump, you can press the palms of your hands across your breasts or cross your arms across your breasts; this pressure on your breasts will stop the flow of your milk. To prevent chapping and possible yeast, moms should keep breast pads inside her bra and change them when damp. I recommend using a LilyPatz, a soft, non-absorbent, flexible, breathable nursing pad that applies pressure, like a finger, on your nipples to stop breast milk from leaking. LilyPadz is made of silicone and can be washed with mild soap and water. These pads are very economical; one pair can last 1-3 months. To prevent wasting your precious breast milk, you can use milk savers to collect breast milk leaking from your opposite breast as you are breastfeeding. Some examples of milk savers are Haakaa, Medela, or Milkies.

In the next chapter, I will discuss a challenge for the breastfeeding mother, returning to work or school.

---

21 Mohrbacher Nancy, 2010 Breastfeeding Answers Made Simple. A Guide Helping Mothers. Amarillo, TX, Hale Publishing.

Chapter 9:

Returning to Work or School

Let's talk about a serious subject for all new moms, returning to work or school. At this time, a mother's primary concern is to have an adequate milk supply for the babysitter and time for pumping at work. My advice for returning to work is planning. When you are preparing to return to work, you need to realize you are only making enough breast milk for your baby. The goal is to increase the milk supply for the babysitter when you return to work. As we have previously discussed, the milk-making hormone from your brain, prolactin, has to increase for adequate milk production. To raise the prolactin level, you need to increase your breast stimulation by increasing the frequency of pumping your breasts; think of your pump as your second baby. Your brain knows no difference between the stimulation to the breasts by your baby or your breast pump.

Let's start planning to go back to work. First, you need to arrange with your employer when and where you can pump. Remind your employer of the amendment to section 7 of the Fair Labor Standards Act (FLSA), which requires employers to provide reasonable break time and a private room for an employee to express breast milk for her child for one year. Mom, you will also need to interview babysitters that do not mind giving and handling breast milk. A big concern when you return to work is your baby taking a bottle. My recommendation is to introduce your baby to a bottle around three weeks of age. A baby sucks differently from a bottle with his tongue and jaw movements. If a baby is introduced to both breast and bottle around three weeks old, he will adapt to both; this is especially important for the mother who has to return to work or school 5-6 weeks after birth. A baby that can drink from breast or bottle decreases the stress for mom, baby, and babysitter.

When should you begin this process of extra pumping to increase your breast milk for returning to work? You need to be aware that prolactin will take weeks, not days, to rise from additional stimulation to your breasts from pumping. Keep in mind your breasts are only producing enough breast milk for one baby. When you are pumping, be patient, do not stop pumping if you see no milk or little milk. At this time, you are not pumping for breast milk; you are pumping to increase prolactin, which will increase your milk supply. When your baby is around three weeks old, start pumping for 15-20 minutes after each feeding in the daytime. Continue this pumping schedule until you are pumping the required ounces of breast milk you need for your individual needs; the amount of required breast milk will vary with every baby and the mother's work routine. If you are working 8 hours a day, you will need to provide your babysitter with 3-4 bottles a day; since the baby usually feeds around every 2-3 hours. On average, a six-week-old baby is drinking about 6 ounces per feeding. If your baby is drinking 6 ounces per feeding every 3 hours or 6 ounces per feeding every 4 hours, you will need to pump 18 to 24 ounces a day for the babysitter. If you are working 8 hours a day and your baby is drinking 6 ounces per feeding, you will need to provide your babysitter with 3-4 bottles containing 6 ounces of breast milk. The key to making extra breast milk is patience and time. I know what you are thinking; *you will not have time at work for the pumping needed to maintain your milk supply.*

I want to put your mind at ease; 100 minutes of breast stimulation between your baby breastfeeding and you pumping your breasts over 24 hours is usually sufficient for maintaining milk supply, as per Stanford Children's Hospital. The 100 minutes of breast stimulation can be in any increments of time between breastfeeding and pumping. Every mother has different schedules for work or school. An example of a breastfeeding and pumping routine, when returning to work, is for you is to breastfeed two times a day for 20 minutes and pump three times a day for 20 minutes. The increments of time between pumping and breastfeeding can be 5 minutes, 10 minutes, or 20 minutes, as long as it is a total of 100 minutes of breast stimulation in 24 hours. Every mother is unique and special; 100 minutes of breast stimulation between your baby breastfeeding and pumping your breasts in 24 hours is a baseline. I want you to experiment with your magic number of minutes you need to pump in 24 hours to produce your required extra milk supply for returning to work; it will take 3-4 weeks to assess the necessary amount of pumping you will need.[22] [23]

Now let's talk about reasons to collect or pump your breast milk; these reasons vary from mother to mother. Pumping is used when a mother returns to work or school, engorgement, flat or inverted nipples, poor or ineffective latch, sleepy baby, or inadequate milk supply. Pumping may be needed for a medical problem with mom, a sick baby in NICU, or prematurity.

How does a breast pump work? A breast pump works as a vacuum or suction, causing a let-down of the breast milk from the milk-making cells deep inside the breast, through the milk ducts, and out the nipple, removing milk from the breast. A breast pump uses gravity for the expressed milk to be collected in a bottle or a freezer bag. The suction power of a breast pump is measured in millimeters (mm) of Mercury, the standard unit for measuring vacuum pressure. A breast pump is made to mimic the baby's sucking pattern. The breast pump needs to have a vacuum or suction of 250 to 300 millimeters of mercury. The pump creates a suction and release cycle that mimics a baby sucking and then slowing down to mimic a baby

22 Lawrence Ruth A. Robert Lawrence 2015 Breastfeeding A Guide Medical Professionals ELSEVIER MOSBY, Philadelphia, Pennsylvania Page 503

23 Walker, Matsha Breastfeeding Management for the Clinician 2nd edition Jones and Barlett Publishers Sudbury, Massachusetts 2011 Page 391

swallowing; this is called a two-phase cycle, 40-60 cycles per minute, one pull per second, which mimics baby sucking at the breast.

How do you pump? When you are pumping, you will place a cone-shaped flange, or nipple shield over the nipple onto the areola or the brown area surrounding the nipple. The suction of the pump pulls the nipple into the tunnel of the flange as milk is expressed. During pumping, the nipples must not rub against the sides of the tunnel of the flange, causing friction and irritation to the nipples. If the pump's flange does not fit correctly, breast milk will not be adequately removed from your milk ducts.

What kind of breast pump should you purchase; this depends on your individual needs. Are you going back to work or staying home? How many days or hours a day will you be working? If you are returning to work, you will need an automatic or double electric breast pump that is lightweight, portable, and effective. If you are going to stay home or need a small amount of pumped milk, a manual, mini-electric, or battery-operated breast pump will be sufficient. Let's take a look at your options for breast pumps.

- Hospital-grade breast pumps are larger and have a stronger motor, ideal for mothers who deliver a premature baby or a sick baby. Mothers can rent a hospital-grade breast pump through the hospital; these pumps are sterilized between moms. Hospital-grade breast pumps mimic the baby's normal sucking rhythm of 40-60 cycles per minute with a suction rate of 300 to 350 millimeters of mercury. Some examples of hospital-grade pumps are Medela Symphony, Lactina, Classic, and Ameda Elite.

- Manual (hand-powered), Mini -electric, or battery-operated pumps allow the mother to pump one breast at a time. These pumps are small, portable, inexpensive, have limited suction, and cycle slowly. These breast pumps are perfect for an occasional bottle. Examples of manual, mini-electric, or battery-operated breast pumps are Medela Harmony (hand-operated), Ameda (hand-operated), Gently Expression (battery, small mini electric), Medela Mini Electric (battery, small mini electric), and the Medela Swing (battery, small mini electric).

- A double electric breast pump is recommended for a mother returning to work. These pumps can be used as a single or double pump. The best double electric breast pumps mimic a baby's sucking and have a two-phase cycle, 40-60 cycles per minute (one pull per second), with a suction rate of 250 to 300 millimeters of mercury. When choosing a double electric breast pump, consider choosing one that has a closed system. A closed pump system has a barrier between the milk collection kit, tubing, and the motor. The closed- system is more hygienic, preventing milk from entering the suction tubing or motor, and preventing air impurities from entering the pumped milk. Examples of closed-system breast pumps include Ameda Purely Yours, Spectra, Lansinoh, and Hygeia.

To spend more time with your baby or if you have limited time for pumping at work, I recommend using an adapter that connects to your breast pump and collects your milk directly into a breast milk storage bag for freezing. Adaptors are available with each type of breast pump.

A pump that may help a working mother is a hands-free breast pump, worn inside your nursing bra. This breast pump has multiple flange sizes available for comfort and effectiveness. These pumps have many advantages for the working mother; it is lightweight and portable, allowing mothers to pump anywhere, such as your desk or car. Another advantage of a hands-free breast pump is that you can pump in any position without spilling. A hands-free breast pump motor is very quiet as you are pumping; this allows you to be on a conference call or sitting at your desk. Some examples of hands-free breast pumps are the Willow, Elvie, and Freemie collection cups.

Hands-free breast pump bras can be beneficial for any mother. With this bra, you do not have to hold the pump flanges onto your breast. The hands–free breast pump bra has a slit or opening in the bra's fabric, keeping the pump's flanges onto your breasts. Using a hands-free breast pump bra allows you to care for other children, read, talk on the phone, or work on your computer. Some examples of hands-free bras are Dairy Fairy and Simple Wishes.

Let's talk about cleaning your breast pump. Why do you think it is essential to wash the parts of your breast pump? Remember that bacteria and mold can grow on your breast pump parts in contact with breast milk or your breasts. I know what you are thinking; *I am exhausted and do not have time to sanitize my breast pump after each pumping.* The good news is you only need to sanitize the washable parts of your breast pump before your first use. According to the FDA, you should boil your breast pump parts for 5-10 minutes before the first use, separating the parts of the pump you will sanitize. Read your breast pump instruction manual for cleaning. After pumping, rinse pump parts with cold water, which removes milk protein residue before washing. Wash pump parts in a clean sink using hot water with detergents that remove milk residue and are non-toxic and hypoallergenic. Clean all pump parts with a cloth or brush and then air-dry pump parts on a clean towel or a drying rack. Do not forget to sanitize bottles, nipples, lids, and brushes. The larger pump parts, such as bottles and flanges, can go on the top rack of your dishwasher. Verify with your breast pump instruction manual which parts of the pump are dishwasher safe. Breast pump tubing should never be immersed in water; wipe off the external or outside of the tubing if needed. Before and after pumping, check your tubing for moisture or mold. If you see mold inside of your breast pump tubing, it should be thrown away and replaced. Call your breast pump manufacturer if you see milk or moisture inside the tubing. If you need a nap or a mental rest, rinse the pump parts that came into contact with your breasts or breast milk with cold water and air dry. Wash the pump parts in hot soapy water after your nap. According to the

FDA, Quick Clean wipes or Quick Clean Microwavable Steam Bags are adequate to disinfect the pump parts used by a single mother, but not for multiple mothers.

Every mother has heard rumors or horror stories about pumping, so let me ease your worries. Pumping should not be painful. So why do mothers complain about pain when they are pumping their breasts? It is important to determine the reason for the pain or discomfort with pumping; so that the cause can be corrected.

All mothers are anxious to make milk for their babies and think they will make more milk if they pump on a high setting. Pumping on high for a prolonged period will cause trauma to your nipples and areola, resulting in pain.

One of the main reasons for sore nipples when pumping your breasts is a poor latch. If you have sore nipples from a poor latch, you need to schedule an appointment with a lactation consultant for evaluation.

Some moms feel pain with pumping from friction around the flange's horn that fits onto the areola of your breast. Before pumping, to reduce friction, apply breast milk or lanolin around the horn's complete circumference. As we have previously discussed, every breast, size of nipples, and areolas are different. Some moms have small areolas, while other moms have large ones. When you are pumping, your nipples should move freely inside the tunnel of the flange. If your nipples rub the inside of the flange tunnel, this indicates the flange is too small, resulting in redness, pain, blisters, and cracking. If you see a large portion of the areola being pulled inside the flange tunnel, the flange is too large for your areola; causing swelling of the areola, pain, and an improper seal around the areola. The flange must fit you correctly to remove the breast milk from your breast adequately. Before you use your breast pump, read the instructions, and evaluate if the flanges fit your areolas correctly; do not wait until the day you need to pump to assess the correct size. If you are having pain with pumping, call the manufacturer of your breast pump. A representative will assist you with choosing a correctly sized flange. You may need two different size flanges, as the areola of your right and left breast may be of different sizes.

An option of flanges that aids in the mother's comfort while pumping is flexible flanges. These angled shaped flanges allow moms to be more comfortable and decrease nipple irritation while pumping. Feeling comfortable and relaxed while pumping your breasts will promote better milk flow.

Women with small breasts and areolas may have a difficult time with a proper fit of their flanges. Flanges made for mothers with small breasts are soft, flexible silicone inserts that fit into a standard 25-millimeter flange. These flanges increase comfort, increase effectiveness of pumping, and increase let-down of the milk

There are times when a mother is uncomfortable and needs to express her breasts, and her baby nor her breast pump is available. You can perform manual or hand expression of your breasts to remove the breast milk in this situation. In preparation for hand expression, you need to wash your hands, sit in a comfortable position, and lead forward to collect the milk (gravity) into a container.

The step-by-step process of performing hand expression
- Place one hand resembling a 'C' shape on your breast
- Your thumb is above the areola, and your index finger is below the areola
- *Press* your thumb and index finger *inward* your chest wall
- *Compress* your breast tissue between your thumb and index finger
- *Roll* your thumb and index finger towards your nipple and *relax*.

When you are rolling your thumb and index finger towards your nipple, do not lift them from your breast. To adequately compress all of the milk ducts, continue moving your index finger and thumb to encircle your entire breast. (Use this system: Using your thumb and index finger Press inward - Compress- Roll and Relax).[24] [25]

A concern when returning to work is freezing and storing breast milk. Pumping takes time and effort, so it is essential to freeze and store your precious breast milk correctly. First, I recommend freezing and storing your milk in amounts you will need for your babysitter; this will vary based on how many days a week and how many hours a day you will be working. When you return to work, you need to be aware that human milk is a food and is not considered a biohazard. Universal precautions are not required when handling human milk, according to The Centers for Disease Control and Prevention (CDC) and the Occupational Safety and Health Administration (OSHA) (See.) Your employer may request that you, as the nursing mom, wipe the area clean with antibacterial wipes after each pumping. Breast milk can be stored in a company refrigerator or the employee's cooler. Always wash your hands before expressing or handling your breast milk. If delivering breast milk to a childcare provider, clearly label the container with the child's name and date. Do not add freshly pumped breast milk to cold milk or frozen milk. After pumping, place milk inside the refrigerator to cool; after milk cools, add it to the refrigerator's previously pumped cold milk. Freeze the cold pumped milk in amounts needed, from 2-6 ounces. It is okay to mix multiple bags of frozen breast milk for feeding. You must always date each container to prevent expiration. Do not save milk from a bottle used during a prior feeding; the baby has suckled on the bottle, and bacteria can grow from the baby's saliva on the nipple and in the milk.

It is essential to be aware of how long your breast milk can be stored at room temperature, refrigerator, and freezer. Breast milk should be kept

---

24 Lauwers,. Judith, BA, IBCLC, FILCA and Swisher , Anna MBA, IBCLC Counseling the Nursing Mother, A Lactation's Consultant Guide 4th edition Jones and Bartlett LEARNING Sudbury, MA 2011 Page 507

25 Lauwers,. Judith, BA, IBCLC, FILCA and Swisher , Anna MBA, IBCLC Counseling the Nursing Mother, A Lactation's Consultant Guide 4th edition Jones and Bartlett LEARNING Sudbury, MA 2011 Page 507

towards the back of a refrigerator to maintain a constant temperature. Do not store breast milk on the inside doors; the temperature changes intermittently when the door opens, affecting the milk's antibacterial factors.[26]

Following a storage chart for freezing and storing breast milk is vital to protect the nutritional factors, protect the antibacterial factors against viruses and bacteria, prevent bacterial growth in the milk, and prevent wastage of your milk.

Breast Milk Storage Chart: Courtesy of La Leche League International

Freshly Pumped Milk at Room Temperature -	4 hours
Freshly Pumped Milk in the refrigerator -	4 days
Thawed milk in a refrigerator, not warmed	24 hours
Insulated cooler bag -	24 hours
Freezer portion of the refrigerator with separate doors	3-6 months
Deep Freezer -	6-12 months

Mothers need to understand how to thaw their breast milk. When you are thawing your breast milk, check the date on your container, and use your oldest milk to prevent expiration. It is best to thaw frozen breast milk by going from the freezer to the refrigerator overnight. If this is not possible and you need a bottle faster, gradual thawing can be performed by swirling the breast milk container in a bowl of warm water. You can also place the container of frozen breast milk under flowing warm water until milk is thawed, and the chill has been removed. Avoid using a microwave to thaw or heat bottles of breast milk. Heating breast milk in a microwave can destroy nutrients in the breast milk, heat the milk unevenly, and burn the baby's mouth. Do not be concerned if your milk looks separated; it is normal for cream or fat to rise. Do not shake the container, gently swirl

---

26 Mohrbacher Nancy , 2010 Breastfeeding Answers Made Simple. A Guide Helping Mothers. Amarillo, TX, Hale Publishing. Page 459

it until the milk is mixed. It is important to remember that thawed breast milk cannot be re-frozen.

Mothers need to be aware of safe, approved containers to freeze and store breast milk. Breast milk cannot be stored and frozen in any container, avoiding those containing a chemical called bisphenol or BPA. This chemical is found in hard plastics and can affect the production and elimination of natural hormones such as estrogen, causing harm to the baby's health. It is best to avoid bottles that contain BPA and are stamped with the numbers 3, 6, and 7. Safe containers recommended for freezing and storing your breast milk that is BPA free are stamped with numbers 2, 4, or 5. There are multiple containers for freezing and storing your breast milk, such as bags, bottles, and glass. Let's review the pros and cons of each container.

- Breast milk storage bags are convenient, disposable, and protect the nutritional properties of the milk. When you purchase storage bags, verify they are BPA free. When freezing and storing your breast milk, avoid using bottle liners and sandwich bags; they are thin and tear easily. Store the breast milk storage bag inside a freezer bag and lay flat to prevent tearing. Do not fill the storage bag to the top since breast milk expands, and the bag will burst if overfilled. An advantage of storage bags is that the milk will thaw faster than other storage containers.

- Plastic breast milk storage bottles are reusable and freezer safe. Verify that the breast milk storage bottles are BPA Free. Storage bottles are less likely to leak compared to storage bags unless they are overfilled. Some examples of breast milk storage bottles are Medela, Lansinoh, Ameda, Snappies, and Spectra wide-mouth bottles.

- Glass containers never contain BPA, lose fewer protective factors, and are reusable and recyclable. Glass containers are breakable; verify your glass container can withstand freezing temperatures without breaking. When using glass containers, thaw the breast milk slowly in the refrigerator overnight to prevent the glass from breaking. Some examples of glass containers are Matyz Glass bottles, Natursutten, Bernardini, and Lifefactory.[27]

- Stainless steel containers should never be used for human milk storage. Dry ice is also hazardous and should never be used in coolers for transporting frozen milk; it gives off carbon dioxide.[28] If traveling, frozen gel packs in a cooler will maintain the milk at a sufficiently cold temperature to minimize bacterial growth for up to 24 hours.[29] When using an insulated cooler bag, the bag should be sealed, and the ice packs should be in contact with the breast milk.

I want to let you be aware of human milk banking. If you are unable to breastfeed or unable to produce adequate breast milk, an option to give your baby breast milk is using donor breast milk. It is recommended to use pasteurized donor human milk from a donor milk bank. The Human Milk Banking Association of Northern America (HMBANA) is an organization that believes all infants should have access to human milk through the support of breastfeeding and the use of pasteurized donor human milk.

If you cannot breastfeed or fully breastfeed, please do not think you are less of a mother. For centuries there have been mothers who could not breastfeed. For that reason, women used wet nurses (a woman who breast-fed babies of other mothers).

I want you to be aware that you can be your own wet nurse using a supplemental nursing system (SNS), a container that can be filled with formula or pasteurized donor human milk. The SNS works by having the milk flow from the container through thin tubes placed alongside your

---

27 Mohrbacher Nancy, 2010 Breastfeeding Answers Made Simple. A Guide Helping Mothers. Amarillo, TX, Hale Publishing. Page 465

28 Mohrbacher Nancy, 2010 Breastfeeding Answers Made Simple. A Guide Helping Mothers. Amarillo, Tx, Hale Publishing. Page 466

29 Hamosh M., Ellis LA., Pollock DR, Henderson TR, Hamosh P: Pediatrica 1996: Breastfeeding and The Working Mother. Effects Time and Temperature Short Term Storage and Bacterial Growth Milk

nipples with adhesive material. There are multiple advantages to using an SNS system; your baby receives milk as he is stimulating your breasts for milk production, and he is becoming more secure at the breast. The SNS system can also be beneficial for an adoptive mother; this enables her to put her baby to the breast using formula or pasteurized donor human milk.

Many mothers only want to pump and give their baby pumped breast milk in a bottle. These mothers tell me they were made to feel inadequate by other mothers and lactation consultants. The only difference in giving a baby pumped breast milk in a bottle versus latching baby onto the breast is that the baby's lips are not on the breast. If the mother wants skin-to-skin, she can remove her shirt and the baby's clothes down to the diaper as with breastfeeding. If a mother decides to breastfeed her baby or give her baby pumped milk via a bottle, that should be the mother's choice without criticism.

Pumping your breasts takes planning and organization. Be kind to yourself, as returning to work or school is stressful and exhausting. Making time for resting and eating can be difficult when you return to work or school. Consider frequent, small, nutritious snacks throughout the day to prevent low blood sugar, increase your energy, and avoid fatigue. In the next chapter, I will discuss how diet and medications can affect breastfeeding.

Chapter 10:

Diet and Medication in Breastfeeding

Moms have told me they are fearful of the possibility of eliminating foods they enjoy eating if they breastfeed. You do not have to eat a perfect diet to make and provide your baby with quality breast milk. As adults, when we eat any food, there is a possibility of a reaction or intolerance to that food; and babies are no different. When you breastfeed you do not have to avoid foods you enjoy, but you want to observe your baby for any signs of a reaction or intolerance to foods you eat. A baby will usually have a reaction or intolerance to food within 12-24 hours after you have eaten that particular food. If your baby is unusually fussy, has increased gas, develops a rash or eczema, has increased spitting up, or cannot sleep, he could be reacting to what you have eaten. Some foods, such as eggs, nuts, or dairy, can cause fussiness, eczema, spitting up, and failure to gain adequate weight, bloody stools, diaper rash, or respiratory symptoms such as wheezing or congestion. The primary allergen for babies is the protein in milk called bovine. Some mothers have to remove foods containing dairy from their diets until they wean their baby from the breast. If your baby has any signs of a reaction or intolerance to a food, please consult with your pediatrician. Do not compare your baby to other babies when you hear stories concerning diet reactions from other mothers and babies. All moms and babies are different.[30] [31]

As a breastfeeding mother, you need to eat an extra 500[32] calories per day to maintain your milk supply and energy level. You do not need to count calories; eat until you satisfy your appetite. The secret for all moms, whether breastfeeding or bottle-feeding, is to eat a balanced diet of fruits, vegetables, and adequate protein to help you feel better physically and mentally. Breastfeeding mothers should drink when you are thirsty and eat when you are hungry. A breastfeeding mother does not need to drink extra fluids to make milk.

You do not have to remove caffeine from your diet while breastfeeding; moderation is the key. It is recommended that breastfeeding mothers consume no more than 300 milligrams of caffeine or 2-3 cups of coffee (470 to 710 milliliters) per day. Caffeine builds up in a baby's body, and the baby cannot eliminate it as quickly as an adult. The build-up of caffeine in a baby's body may cause the baby to be fussy, irritable, or be unable to sleep.[33]

Does breastfeeding mean you cannot have an occasional alcoholic drink? Breastfeeding mothers can drink alcoholic beverages but need to wait 2 hours after each alcoholic drink before breastfeeding. To decrease the amount of alcohol absorbed into your bloodstream, have your alcoholic beverage with a meal. Another option is to pump your breasts and then pour your breast milk down the drain that contains alcohol (pump and dump); give your baby a bottle of pumped breast milk or formula.[34]

---

30 Pearson Glaze Philippa IBCLC: Breastfeeding Support Article Name Elimination Diet November 2019

31 Pearson Glaze Philippa IBCLC: Breastfeeding Support Article Name Elimination Diet November 2019

32 Riodan and Wambach Breastfeeding and Human Lactation 4th edition Jones and Bartlett Publishers, Sudbury, Massachusetts 2010 page 498

33 Jacobson Hilary Mother Food and Herbs that Promote Milk Production and a Mother's Health Rosalind Press Lexington Kentucky 2004 Page 113

34 Biancuzzo Maria , Breastfeeding the Newborn, Clinical Strategies for Nurses Mosby, Herdon Virginia 1999 Page 72

Fish is a good source of protein and an excellent DHA source, omega-three fatty acid, which improves the baby's visual and brain development. It is essential to limit fish to 2 servings or 12 ounces a week due to mercury levels. Fish low in mercury are salmon, pollock, catfish, cod, clams, haddock, scallops, lobster, shrimp, and canned light tuna (canned albacore has higher mercury, limit to 6 ounces a week). It is recommended to avoid shark, king mackerel, tilefish, and swordfish.[35]

Breastfeeding mothers who are vegetarians can support their babies' growth and development if mom is well nourished. The mother needs to have a balanced diet of grains, legumes, nuts, fruits, and fats. Her diet needs to include protein and calcium sources, such as eggs, seeds, beans, cereals, soy, and dark green leafy vegetables. These mothers need to be aware that the primary source of vitamin B12 is in animal protein, such as meat, fish, poultry, eggs, and dairy. A deficiency of vitamin B12 can cause a baby to develop irritability, feeding problems, and low muscle tone. It is important vegetarian breastfeeding mothers discuss their diet with their ob-gyn for the possibility of taking vitamin B12 supplements.[36] www.mypyramid.gov/ my pyramid/breastfeeding

Breast milk is low in vitamin D; it is needed for your baby's bone development and immune system.[37] Research shows maternal supplementation of 6400 IU (international units) of vitamin D per day will supply the nursing infant with his needed vitamin D amounts. Discuss vitamin D supplementation with your pediatrician. [38]

35 Mahak Arora Article Name Eating Fish During Breastfeeding, Is It Safe? July 10 2018 Dr Alexander Laith ABC News Article Name FDA extols virtues of fish for pregnant and breastfeeding mothers July 3 2019

36 Lauwers Judith and Swisher Anna Counseling the Nursing Mother 5th edition Jones and Bartlett Learning Sudbury, Massachusetts 2011 Page 427-428 Mohrbacher Nancy, Breastfeeding Answers Made Simple, A Guide for Helping Mothers Hale Publishing Amarillo, Texas 2010 Page 523-524

37 Adams, Helen Article: Medical University South Carolina. Name article: Vitamin D research leads to first of its kind recommendation for pregnant patients. May 4, 2017

38 Dr Hollis Bruce : Article , Maternal Verses Infant Vitamin D Supplantation During Lactation Pediatrics October 2015

Believe it or not, your breast milk color and taste can change when you eat or drink certain foods and beverages. Your breast milk may have a yellow or green tint from foods are beverages you consume. Do not be concerned; the milk is safe for your baby. Your breast milk's normal color can range from clear, cream, white, or have a blue hue. If you eat various flavors when you breastfeed, your baby will be familiar with these flavors when you introduce solid foods.

Mothers need to be aware that most medications are safe and compatible with breastfeeding, depending on the levels found in breast milk. Doctors can refer to LACTMED or *Medication and Mothers Milk* by Dr. Thomas Hale, PhD. to verify how much, if any, of the medication enters the breast milk and how long the medication stays in the breast milk. If you are prescribed a medication, verify it is safe to take while breastfeeding with your ob-gyn. Do not pump your breasts and then pour your breast milk down the drain until you have consulted with your physician. [39] [40]

The first few weeks after birth, you will not have an appetite. Please do not focus on eating three meals a day; instead, snack on healthy snacks every 2-3 hours to keep your energy level elevated. I suggest having a bowl of healthy snacks near you at all times, such as trail mix, vegetables, seeds, oats, nuts, or grains. Munching on healthy snacks throughout the day will help your body heal and promote your physical and mental health.

All babies do not look the same at birth. Newborns may have different changes on the surface of their skin or reactions from mothers' hormones. In the next chapter, I will discuss your newborn's normal characteristics and increase your knowledge of caring for your baby.

---

39 Hale Thomas Medications and Mother's Milk 14th edition Hale Publishing Amarillo, Texas 2010 Page 5

40 Berlin, Chester American Academy Pediatrics: The Transfer of Drugs and Other Chemicals into Human Milk Pediatrics Vol 93 January 1994

Chapter 11:

Normal Physical Characteristics and Care of the Newborn

Let's talk about normal physical characteristics you may notice on your newborn. First, I want you to remember every baby is different in appearance, personality, and developmental stages. Newborns are small and delicate, making mothers feel anxious and fearful to hold, feed, and care for them. To decrease your fear and anxiety, I want to increase your knowledge by discussing your newborn's normal physical appearances, normal reflexes, and the development of your baby's sense of sight and hearing. We will also review how to bottle-feed your baby and how to burp your baby. Mothers are always concerned that they will not understand their baby's needs; your baby will voice his needs to you with different cries. We will discuss multiple reasons your baby may cry to meet a particular need. Day by day, you will learn his different types of cries.

Let's review normal physical appearances you may notice on your newborn.

- Acrocyanosis: At birth, your newborn may have blue hands and feet; this is normal and does not mean your baby has a disease or is cold. When a baby is born, a large percentage of oxygen in their blood flows to their brain, heart, lungs, kidneys, and other vital organs, and less oxygen in their blood flows to their hands and feet. Within a few days to a week, the baby's blood vessels open wider, and the color of their hands and feet change to a pinker hue.

- Mongolian spots: Babies born of darker-skinned parents may have areas on their bodies that appear blue-gray. These irregular shaped, bruised-looking regions are caused by the pigment not making its way to the surface of the baby's skin. Mongolian spots can be located anywhere on your baby's body; they are not tender to the touch, they are not birthmarks, and they do not reveal a disease. Mongolian spots slowly disappear when your child is around five years old.

- Blood vagina: Mothers should not panic if they see a scant amount of blood from the vagina of their baby girls. Hormones from the mother can cause swelling around the baby's vagina and cause intermittent drops of blood from your baby's vagina. As maternal hormones decrease, swelling around your baby's vagina and bloody spotting from your baby's vagina will resolve within a few weeks.

- Swollen breasts: Both baby boys and baby girls may have swollen, lumpy areas on their breasts, and their breasts may leak drops of milk; caused by the mother's hormones. Your baby's breasts may be tender, so be gentle when cleaning. After a few weeks, when maternal hormones decrease, these symptoms will resolve.

- Soft spots (fontanels): During delivery, the bones on your baby's head overlap or mold for your baby to come through the birth canal or vagina. After birth, the bones are separated; these open, soft separations are called fontanels. The posterior, triangle-shaped, softened area in the back of the baby's head will meet and fuse when your baby is around six weeks of age. The anterior, kite-shaped, softened area will meet and fuse when your baby is approximately 18 months old.

- Vernix: At birth, your baby may have vernix or a white, sticky, or cheese-like material noted in the creases of his arms, legs, groin, and neck. In utero, this vernix coating covers your baby's entire body as it moistures and protects the baby's skin. During delivery, the vernix's waxy feel can assist the baby in sliding through the vagina or birth canal. Within a few days to a week, the vernix will gradually disappear.

- Lanugo: I do not want you to be shocked when you may see you're newborn covered in short, black hairs, mostly on his arms, legs, and back. These short, soft hairs grow on your baby's skin in utero and help the cheesy vernix stay on the baby's skin for protection. These lanugo hairs will begin to fall off before delivery or within a few weeks after birth.

- Milia: Newborns may have tiny, white bumps on their nose, cheeks, or chin; these white bumps are called milia. Please do not attempt to pop or rub them off; they are not whiteheads or acne development. Milia are caused by oil forming under the skin; they will resolve or disappear in a few weeks after birth.

You might not be aware that newborns have many normal reflexes. Let's discuss some reflexes of your newborn to increase your knowledge and decrease any anxiety you may have if you observe your baby demonstrating these reflexes.

- Hiccups: Involuntary spasms of the diaphragm (a dome-shaped muscle that separates your abdomen from your chest). Hiccups are normal and are not uncomfortable for your baby.

- Sneezing: Your baby breathes through his nose for the first six months of his life. Breathing through his nose allows lint or dust to irritate the lining of his nose, causing the baby to sneeze. Sneezing does not mean your baby is sick.

- Startle or Moro Reflex: A normal reflex of your baby's reaction or response to loud noises. When your baby hears a loud noise, he will spread out his arms and then pull his arms inward; he may or may not cry. Within 4-6 months, as your baby becomes more secure in his new environment, he will have fewer startle reflexes.

- Palmer Reflex: Occurs when you stroke the palm of your newborn's hand and his fingers close; this makes mommy feel good that her baby is holding her hand.

- Rooting Reflex: Is an indication that your newborn is still hungry; he will root and turn his head when his cheek or lip is touched

When can your baby hear and see?
- Hearing: In utero, your baby can hear your muffled voice and music; this is why your baby turns his head when he hears your voice. Before you are discharged from the hospital, your baby will have a newborn hearing screening test.

- Vision: Your baby can see around 8-10 inches at birth. When you are bonding and talking to your baby, hold him close to your face so he can see his beautiful mommy. Do not be concerned if your baby's eyes appear crossed; this will decrease as his eyes become stronger and more coordinated. You can help to coordinate his eyes by playing with a rattle and moving the rattle from side to side. Talk, sing, and smile to your baby, and within a few weeks, you will notice how your baby will begin to look at your face. When he is around 6-12 weeks old, he will be smiling back at you.

We forget at birth; your baby is a blank slate. This world is new to him. You and your support person are his role models; he will listen, watch, and mimic you. Making eye contact, talking, and touching your baby can play a big part in his development. It is essential to play with your baby, but independent playtime is critical in teaching your baby to self- soothe. If you hold your baby all day, he will expect to be held all day, resulting in mom feeling exhausted, frustrated, and overwhelmed. Your support person will come home from work, finding you still in your PJ's and crying, "I cannot even take a shower." When your baby can independently play and self-soothe, it allows you to have mommy downtime, decreasing your stress. To develop independent play and self-soothing, place your baby in a baby swing, bouncy seat, or floor time (tummy time), starting when he comes home from the hospital. I would intermittently use the swing, bouncy seat, or tummy time throughout the day when your baby is awake. Be aware that for the first 1-2 weeks after birth, tummy time, swinging, or bouncy seat may only last 2-5 minutes; your baby has to adjust to his new world. Day by day, your baby will begin to love being on the floor, in the bouncy seat, or a swing as his head, neck, back, and stomach become stronger. Independent play and self-soothing will decrease your baby's stress at daycare or with a baby sitter when you return to work around 5-6 weeks after delivery.

"My baby will not take a bottle; I do not know what to do. I have to return to work in 2 weeks."

I have heard mothers express this stressed, desperate statement multiple times. Let's discuss what you can do to prevent your baby from refusing a bottle. When your baby refuses to take a bottle, it creates stress and frustration for you and your baby. All bottle companies claim their nipples are comparable to the breast, decreasing nipple confusion for the baby. Every baby is unique and sucks differently. Just because one bottle company claims their nipples reduce nipple confusion, making it easier for a baby to transition to a bottle, does not mean every baby will like their nipples. Slow-flow nipples, appropriate to the baby's age, are best for preventing the baby from choking and gagging. I recommend starting one bottle at bedtime when your baby is around three weeks of age; if you wait until your baby is 4-5 weeks old, the majority of babies will refuse to drink from a bottle.

We have to be practical, your baby has only breastfed since birth, and we cannot expect him to accept and drink from a plastic nipple immediately. If your baby refuses to drink from a bottle, introducing a bottle should be slow, not stressful, or forceful. First, try a 4-ounce bottle with the nipple you desire to use and let the baby play with it like a toy. Intermittently gently place the nipple at the baby's lips; using your fingers, compress the nipple to squirt a little milk onto your baby's lips. After a few days of using this maneuver, have your support person offer your baby a bottle with warm milk at bedtime. Babies can smell their mommy and sometimes will not immediately accept a bottle from you. Another method to help your baby take a bottle is Dream- Feeding your baby. To perform the dream-feeding method, breastfeed your baby before you go to bed. Your baby will be very sleepy, as he is breastfeeding; since he has been sleeping for a few hours. Breastfeed your baby for around 5 minutes and then gently and slowly place the nipple of a bottle into your baby's mouth; your baby will suck on the nipple in a sleepy state. Bottle-feed your baby 1-2 ounces of warmed pumped milk or formula. Dream-feeding is a win-win situation; the baby is becoming comfortable bottle-feeding. Another positive result of the dream -feeding method is the baby's stomach becoming full; this results in baby sleeping longer and mommy sleeping longer.[41]

When your baby can alternate being fed from breast to bottle effectively, stress is reduced for baby, mother, and baby sitter. There is a large variety of bottles and nipples on the market. Every baby is different; you may have to try multiple bottles and nipples for your baby. Some examples of bottles that your baby may accept and drink from: Calma by Medela, MAM, Adair, Comotomo, Dr. Brown Natural Flow Wide Neck, Tommee Tippee, and Munchkin.

---

41 Karp Harvey MD Article Name: What Is Dream Sleeping? And How to Dream Feed? May 28, 2020

A mother has to learn how to bottle-feed her baby; just like a mother has to learn how to breastfeed her baby. There are multiple kinds of formulas on the market, including milk-based, soy-based, and protein-based. Specific formulas, Nutramigen and Alimentum, are used for colic and allergies. Formulas come in ready to feed, liquid concentrate, or powder that needs to be mixed with purified water or distilled water. When bottle-feeding, I recommend using the Pace Bottle-Feeding Method. When using the Pace Bottle-Feeding Method, feed your baby in an upright or a sitting position, hold the bottle horizontal, tickle the baby's lips with the nipple of the bottle, and the baby will latch onto the nipple. After your baby sucks on the bottle for a few minutes, lower the bottle to allow your baby to swallow and rest. Feed your baby until he is content, happy, and showing no hunger or feeding cues; every baby is different. When you bottle-feed, avoid propping your bottle or leading the bottle against a blanket or a pillow. When you prop a bottle, your baby may suck air into his stomach or choke on the milk. Feeding time, breastfeeding or bottle-feeding, is a time to hold, talk, bond, and enjoy your baby.

How much pumped milk or formula should you feed your baby? We need to remember that every baby is different; feed your baby per his feeding cues. The first week after birth, your formula-fed newborn may drink around 1-2 ounces of formula per feeding; on average, your bottle-fed baby will eat around every 2-3 hours.[42] Babies will gradually increase the amount of milk they need, per each baby's feeding cues, such as fussiness or hand-mouth activity. As documented in an article, The Fed Is Best Foundation, stomach emptying is continuous, which allows for the possibility of an increase in the amount of milk needed per each baby's stomach. A baby will tell you when he is hungry by his feeding cues, and he will tell

---

42 Altman, Tanya MD Caring for your baby and young child to age 5. 7th edition. 2019 American Academy Pediatrics Bantam Books New York New York page 87

you when his stomach is full by becoming limp, relaxed, and showing no feeding cues.[43]

Let's talk about burping when you assist your baby to release air from his stomach. Your baby may develop air in his stomach when he drinks fast, cries, and swallows air. The air entering your baby's stomach can cause abdominal pain and spitting up, resulting in your baby being fussy and irritable. Mothers can assist the baby to release air from his stomach by performing different burping positions. A bottle-fed baby swallows more air than a breastfeeding baby; the mother should attempt to burp her baby 2-3 times during the feeding to decrease air entering the baby's stomach. Breastfed babies swallow less air but still need to be burped when rotating breasts. Multiple mothers have asked me, "How do I burp my baby." I have described some burping positions that may be beneficial for you.

- The most common burping position is the upright position with your baby's body vertically against your chest. In this burping position, your baby's head is on your shoulder. Place one of your hands on the baby's bottom for support while using your opposite hand to pat or rub your baby's back.

- The football hold for burping can be helpful when your baby is fussy. Place your baby's stomach face down on your forearm, supporting baby's chin with your fingers, with his legs straddled between your forearm. In the football burping position, rock your forearm, intermittently patting the baby on his back with your opposite hand. Babies love the rocking motion, which may be helpful when your baby has signs of gas, pulling his legs up to his chest and crying.

- Another burping position is positioning your baby's stomach horizontally across your legs while patting him on his back. In

---

43 THE NEWBORN STOMACH SIZE MYTH IT'S NOT 5-7 ML Jody Daly MS RN IBCLC June 12, 2017

this position, the pressure is being applied to your baby's stomach by your legs, decreasing his abdominal discomfort.

Let's talk about how your baby voices his needs to you. Crying is your baby's only means of communication; your baby is sending you a message. Using your senses of seeing and hearing, you will learn your baby's needs and the different types of cries for his needs. When your baby is hungry, he will cry, remember crying for hunger is his last hunger cue. Your baby has already given you multiple cues for hunger, including hand-mouth activity or playing with his tongue. Your baby may cry if he is having pain or discomfort from gas. Your baby will rub his eyes and be fussy when he's tired; it is nap or bedtime. Your baby will cry if he is too hot or cold; the recommended temperature of your home should be between 68-72 degrees[44] Fahrenheit. When all else fails, check your baby's diaper, he will cry if he is uncomfortable from a wet or dirty diaper. Your baby has multiple needs; love is his number -one need; I recommend lots of kissing and cuddling.

If you cannot find any apparent reason for your baby crying, your baby may have colic? Colic is intense, loud crying that causes your baby to be inconsolable. These crying periods can last 3 hours or more a day; many times are occurring between 6 pm and midnight. Babies from smoking households tend to be fussier and have more colic symptoms.[45] Soothing and calming your baby when he is crying, or upset will decrease stress for both you and your baby. Dr. Harvey Karp, the author of *Happiest Baby on the Block*, has written techniques to reduce crying and fussiness to calm your baby. Let's discuss the effects of swaddling, sucking, white noise, and the use of motion with a swing or bouncy seat for calming and soothing your baby.[46]

---

44 Novak Sara Article Name : What's the Right Temperature for Baby? April 2000

45 Walker, Marsha Breastfeeding Management for the Clinician: Using the Evidence, 2nd edition Jones and Bartlett Publishers Sudbury, Massachusetts 2011 Page 208 - 313

46 Karp Harvey MD Happiest Baby on The Block Bantam Books 2015 New York, New York

- Swaddling soothes and calms your baby, decreasing the startle reflex and increasing sleep. According to Dr. Karp, swaddling is the key to reducing crying and helps the baby sleep on his back. "That's why I recommend swaddling for all babies," Karp said.

- Sucking is a natural need for all babies. This non-nutritive sucking releases endorphins; to aid your baby to sleep. I do not recommend a pacifier to substitute a feeding; you can offer a pacifier after feeding for relaxation.

- Shush is a sound your baby has heard inside your uterus; this sound is similar to the sound of blood flowing through the umbilical cord. Sound machines with white noise, hairdryers, and vacuum cleaners sound similar to the noise inside your baby's home for the last 40 weeks. When he hears these familiar sounds, he will be more relaxed and calm.

- Swinging is very relaxing for a newborn, similar to his active movements in utero in response to his mother's activities. When you bring your baby home from the hospital and place him in a flat crib or cradle that does not move, he will cry; it will take time for your baby to adjust to his new environment. To assist in his adjustment, I recommend placing your baby in a swing or bouncy seat when you arrive home from the hospital. Your baby will slowly adjust and begin to love his swing or bouncy seat; this will entertain your baby, increasing mommy time to relax and rest.

Massage can be a gentle stimulation to calm your baby. When you touch and stroke your baby's skin during massage, endorphins are released and cause your baby to feel calm and relaxed. Massaging your baby's abdominal muscles can help with cramping, gas, and colic. I think the number-one benefit of massaging your baby is the bonding between you and your baby.

Being a parent is the most challenging job you will ever have. I came across these suggestions from the Fairfax (Virginia) County Department of Family Services to increase your child's self-esteem.

- Provide praise and recognition for accomplishments.

- Take their emotions, ideas, and feelings seriously. Do not belittle them.

- Have rules and enforce them.

- Be a good role model.

- Set goals and expectations they can achieve.

- Understand and accept different cultures and values.

- Give your child responsibility, providing them a feeling of being valued.

- Be available to provide support.

- Take an interest in their activities and interests.

- Discuss problems and solutions without placing blame, without attack.

- Build self-esteem: Say Thank you, and that was a great idea.

- Hug them; tell them they are terrific and that you love them.

Remember, there is no perfect parent. You are not a super mom; you are human. Enjoy each moment as your baby reaches each milestone of his life with your guidance, love, and support. When you are breastfeeding, a milestone that can be difficult for mom and baby is weaning baby from breastfeeding to bottle-feeding. In the next chapter, we will discuss when and how to wean your baby from breastfeeding slowly. There comes a time when each mother and baby is ready to wean.

Chapter 12:

Weaning

Let's talk about weaning, when a mother gradually introduces a baby or toddler to another food source, slowly decreasing the amount of time breastfeeding. *When I talk to mothers about weaning, their biggest fear is pain and being uncomfortable.* There are multiple reasons mothers decide to wean their baby or toddler. Each mother has individual life stressors that she has to juggle. Every mother and baby is different, so when a mother decides she wants to start weaning, it should be her decision. There is no right and wrong how long a mother should breastfeed; the length of time a mother breastfeeds depends on her comfort and stress. Juggling life when you breastfeed, returning to work, organizing a pumping schedule, caring for yourself, and caring for your family is hard. Breastfeeding takes a lot of time and effort. When you decide it is time to wean your baby, you want the process to go smoothly with mild discomfort and stress. I *want to ease your mind and decrease your fear of weaning by providing you with some suggestions to reduce pain.*

Let's talk about how and when to start the weaning process. I am going to give you a few examples of ways to wean. Weaning should be a slow, gradual process of decreasing the time you pump your breasts and decreasing breastfeeding frequency, decreasing stress and frustration for mom and baby.

- The first option for weaning is to skip one breastfeeding or pumping session every 3-4 days, taking away daytime sessions first, gradually decreasing the amount of time you pump by 5 minutes every 3-4 days.

  For example, skip a one-morning pumping session every 3-4 days or miss one breastfeeding session in the afternoon every 3-4 days. Continue skipping breastfeeding and pumping sessions in the daytime every 3-4 days, along with decreasing the amount of time you pump by 5 minutes every 3-4 days. Decreasing breastfeeding and pumping will result in a lack of breast stimulation, causing milk supply to decrease gradually.

  The mother should continue to breastfeed at bedtime; babies love the closeness to mommy. Breast milk will gradually dry up, and your baby will decrease the length of time he wants to be at the breast at bedtime.

- The second option for weaning is to decrease the length of time you pump 5 minutes every 3-4 days, according to the mother's pumping schedule. A working mom usually pumps 3-4 times a day. For Example:

  Decrease pumping from 20-15 minutes for 3-4 days.

  Decrease pumping from 15-10 minutes for 3-4 days.

  Decrease pumping from 10-5 minutes for 3-4 days

  Decrease pumping from 5 minutes to 2-3 minutes for 3-4 days.

Continue to allow baby to nurse in the morning, afternoon, and bedtime. Breastfeeding 2-3 times a day and slowly decreasing the length of time you pump will result in a lack of breast stimulation, causing milk supply to decrease gradually. Your baby will begin to have shorter nursing sessions due to a decrease in milk supply.

To assist with decreasing milk supply as you are weaning, I recommend decreasing fluids, sipping on sage or jasmine tea, sucking on a peppermint candy or menthol throat lozenges, and preparing foods that contain parsley. Avoiding nipple stimulation with intercourse and wearing a bra day and night can prevent an increase in your milk supply. If your breasts feel full and uncomfortable, you can take a warm shower with a brief massage, pump your breasts for 3-5 minutes, or briefly hand express your breasts for 3-5 minutes. *If you* gradually remove small amounts of milk from your breast during the weaning process, milk production will slowly decrease, preventing the development of plugged ducts or mastitis. As you decrease breastfeeding and pumping, your brain decreases prolactin production, decreasing your milk supply. Be patient as you are weaning; it may take a few weeks for the milk inside of your milk ducts to dry up. To decrease swelling of your breasts and under your armpits, use bags of frozen vegetables such as corn or peas and washed chilled cabbage leaves inside your bra or breast therapy cold relief packs. Cold or ice treatments can be used for 15-20 minutes, 3-4 times a day, or what time frame is comfortable for you. You can also take ibuprofen for discomfort. Weaning your baby from breast to a bottle is a big adjustment for your baby. I recommend singing to your baby during bottle- feeding and increasing hugs and kisses; decreasing the stress of this transition. Mom, you will also need extra hugs and kisses as your breastfeeding hormones, prolactin, and oxytocin, decrease; causing you to have temporary feelings of sadness for a few weeks.

There are certain times I would not recommend to wean. I will not wean if you or your baby are sick, in times of stress such as moving or changing jobs, when a baby has a growth spurt, or when the baby is teething. I feel weaning during these times would add more stress to both mom and baby. When you decide to wean, congratulate yourself for all the hard work and dedication you have made in breastfeeding your baby

Summary: As you were reading my book, you noticed the repetition of the importance of stimulation of a sleepy newborn and early stimulation to your breasts by your baby breastfeeding or pumping your breasts. This early breast stimulation will promote long-term milk production. Breastfeeding success is dependent on your milk supply.

Conclusion: Breastfeeding is a feeding method for your baby; most important are the physical health of your baby and your physical and mental health as the mother. After delivery, mothers have a hormonal rollercoaster with a drop in their pregnancy hormones, estrogen and progesterone, and a rise in their breastfeeding hormones, oxytocin, and prolactin. These shifts in hormones can cause prolonged excessive crying and sadness; this is a sign of perinatal mood and anxiety disorder. If you have extended sadness, crying, or a decreased interest in caring for yourself or your baby, please ask for help. Do not be embarrassed or ashamed; postpartum support groups are available to provide you with guidance and support.

Enjoy your baby!

References

Adams Helen, Vitamin D Research Leads to 1st in its Kind, Recommendations Pregnant Patients, University South Carolina May 4, 2017

Alexander. Laith, MD ABC News Article Name: FDA Extols Virtues of Fish for Pregnant and Breastfeeding Mothers July 3, 2019

Altman, Tanya MD Caring for Your Baby and Young Child to Age 5 7th editions Bantam Books New York, New York 2019

Berggren, Kirsten, Ph.D., BCLC. *Working without Weaning*. Hale Publishing Amarillo, Texas 2006

Berlin, Chester American Academy Pediatrics: The Transfer of Drugs and Other Chemicals into Human Milk Pediatrics Vol 93 January 1994

Biancuzzo, Marie. Breastfeeding the Newborn Mosby, Herdon, Virginia 1999

Clay, Barbara Wilson, BS, IBCLC, and Kay Hoover Med, IBCLC. 2nd edition Lact News-Press Austin, Texas 2002

Daly, Jody The Newborn's Stomach Size Myth It's Not 5-7 ml June 12. 1017

DeCarvalho M. Robertson S. and Friedman A. Klaus M Effects of frequent breastfeeding on early milk production and infant weight Pediatrics 1983

Fairfax County Department of Family Services: Self-Esteem/Ways to Help Children Like Themselves. Verbal Permission for use

Ferber, S.G. and R Makhoul The effects of skin to skin contact (kangaroo care) shortly after birth on the neurobehavioral responses of the term newborn Pediatrics 2004

Furman L. Minich N., Hack M., Pediatrics 2002: Correlates Lactation in Mothers of very birth weight infants

Glaze, Pearson, Philippa Breastfeeding Support Elimination Diet November 2019

Hale, Thomas W. *Medication in Mothers Milk. Hale Publishing Amarillo, Texas 2012*

Hale, Thomas, and Berens Pamela, MD. *Clinical Therapy in Breastfeeding Patients Hale Publishing Amarillo, Texas 2010*

Hamosh M., Ellis LA., Pollock DR, Henderson TR, Hamosh P: Pediatric 1996: Breastfeeding and The Working Mother. Effects Time and Temperature Short Term Storage and Bacterial Growth Milk

Hanson A. Lars MD Ph.D. IMMUNOBIOLOGY of Human Milk, How Breastfeeding Protects Babies p 167 Pharma soft Publishing Amarillo, Texas 2004

Jacobson, Hilary. 2013 *Mother Food, Foods and herbs that promote milk production and a mother's health Rosalind Press, Lexington, Kentucky*

Hanson a. Lars MD Ph.D. IMMUNOBIOLOGY of Human Milk p 167

Karp, Harvey, MD. 2003. *Happiest Baby on the Block Bantam, Books New York, New York 2015*

Karp Harvey MD What is Dream Sleeping? How Do you Dream Feed? May 28, 2020

Lauwers, Judy, and Anna Swisher. *Counseling the Nursing Mother*. 5th edition Jones & Bartlett Sudbury, Massachusetts 2011

Lawrence, Ruth A., and Robert M Lawrence. *Breastfeeding: A Guide for the Medical Professional*, 7th edition Elsevier Mosby, Philadelphia Pennsylvania 2011

Mahak, Arora Eating Fish During Breastfeeding. Is It Safe? July 2018

May's Ina Guide to Breastfeeding Bantam Books New York, New York 2009

Meek Younger Joan MD NPHD FAAP IBCLC New Mother Guide to Breastfeeding **Bantam** Trade Paperbacks New York, New York 2011

Mohrbacher, Nancy IBCLC FILCA Breastfeeding Answers Made Simple. A Guide for Helping Mothers Hale Publishing Amarillo, Texas 2010

Moran, Elaine. *Bon Appe'tit Baby: You're Breastfeeding Guide.* Treasured Child Publications Freedom, California 2005

Newman, Jack, and Teresa Pittman. *The Latch and Other Keys to Breastfeeding Success.* Hale Publishing Amarillo, Texas 2006

Newman, Jack and Teresa Pitman The Ultimate Breastfeeding Book Of Answers Three Rivers Press New York, New York 2006

Novak, Sara What's the Night Temperature for Baby April 2020

Patel, Sonal Mommy MD Guide to Twins, Triplets and More Momosa Publishing, National Book Network Hellertown, Pennsylvania 2018

Pictures of breastfeeding positions: Written Permission given per parents

Picture of Montgomery Glands: Written Permission from *Coordinator:* Marta Jendra, *Journal Sales Publications,* Radiological Society of North America, Oak Brook, IL 60523

Riordan, Jan, and Karen Wabash. *Breastfeeding and Human Lactation: Fourth edition.*

Jones and Bartlett Publishers Sudbury, Massachusetts 2010

Spangler, Amy, MN, RN, IBCLC. *Breastfeeding: A Parent's Guide 2002 7th edition Amy's Baby Company Atlanta, Georgia* 1995

Tiller, Sue, IBCLC. *Breastfeeding 101.* TLC Publishing Centreville, Virginia 2002

Vector Stock: Permission to use the picture of the anatomy of the breast

Walker, Marsha. *Breastfeeding Management of the Clinician.* 2nd edition Jones and Bartlett Publishers Sudbury, Massachusetts 2016

Washington Post: article with permission

West, Diana IBCLC, and Lisa Marasco M.A. IBCLC. *Making More Milk.* McGraw Hill, New York, New York 2009

Williamson, M., and Murti K.: Effects on storage, time, and temperature composition of containers biologic components of human milk: J Hum Lact 1996

Wright, Nancy, and Kathleen Marinelli and the American Academy of Breastfeeding Medicine ABA Clinical Protocol # 1: Guidelines for Blood Sugar Monitoring and Treatment of Hypoglycemia in Term and Late Preterm Neonates Revised 2014 Volume 9 November 4, 2014

Websites:

Academy of Breastfeeding Medicine website: www.bfmed.org

American Academy of Pediatrics website: www.aap.org

BESTFED.COM website: www.bestfed.com

BREASTFEEDING AFTER BREAST REDUCTION website: www.bfar.org

Fussy Baby: website: www.thefussybaby.com

Fed Is Best Foundation: Non-Profit Organization Breastfeeding and Bottle-Feeding Safety

website: www.fedisbes.org

Human Milk Banking Association of North America (HMBANA) website: www.hmbana.org

International Breastfeeding Center (Dr. Jack Newman Breastfeeding Clinic)

website: ibconline.ca

Canadian Breastfeeding Foundation www.canadianbreastfeedingfounda-tion.ca

Infant Massage USA

Kelly Mom: website www.kellymom.com

La Leche League International: website: www.lalecheleague.org

Mothering Magazine website: www.mothering.com

Perinatal Mood and Anxiety Disorder/Post-Partum Depression websites: www.postpartum.net

www.postpartumprogress.com

UNICEF (United Nations Children's Fund) publications website: www.unicef.org/apublic

Vitamin B 12 for Vegans or Vegetarians Good Tasting Nutritional Yeast

website: www.healthy-eating.com

THE NATIONAL WOMEN'S HEALTH INFORMATION CENTER BREASTFEEDING HELPLINE website: www.4woman.gov

Very Well Family website www.verywellfamily.com

WHO (WORLD HEALTH ORGANIZATION) website: www.who.int